12 RB

D1799576

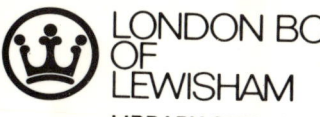 LONDON BOROUGH
OF
LEWISHAM
LIBRARY SERVICE

Author

_____

Title

BOOK STORE

Books or discs must be returned on or before the last date stamped on label or on
card in book pocket. Books or discs can be renewed by telephone, letter or personal
call unless required by another reader. After library hours use the Ansafone
Service (01 - 698 7347). For hours of opening and charges see notices at the
above branch, but note that all lending departments close   . on Wednesday
and all libraries are closed on Sundays, Good Friday, Christmas Day, Bank Holidays
and Saturdays prior to Bank Holidays.

FOOD FIT FOR HUMANS

By the same author

FOOD FOR THE GOLDEN AGE

ART INTO LIFE

ART AS UNDERSTANDING

THE CRYSTALLINE THEME

FRANK AVRAY WILSON

FOOD FIT
FOR HUMANS

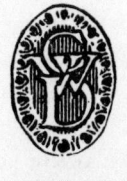

LONDON
THE C. W. DANIEL COMPANY

First published in Great Britain
by The C. W. Daniel Company Limited
60 Muswell Road, London N10 2BE

© Frank Avray Wilson 1975

ISBN 085207 132 9

LEWISHAM LIBRARY SERVICE

	BRANCH	COPY
LBN.		
SBN. 0 85207.132.9	3	
CLASS NUMBER 613.2	CATEGORY	
BOOK-SELLER DEN.	INVOICE DATE 14.3.76	
ACC.	V80707	

Set in eleven on twelve point Baskerville.
Printed by the Northumberland Press Ltd, Gateshead,
and bound by Staples Printers Ltd,
Rochester, Kent, using Dalmore artwork supplied by
Frank Grunfeld Ltd, London.

CONTENTS

1. The Object Defined

Appearance can be deceptive. Who is happy? Who is healthy? Assurances can also be false, like the dictum, 'a little of what you like is good for you'. Even rats, given the chance to eat what they like, eat the wrong things. Sight, smell and taste have been so falsified that the native senses are now powerless to distinguish nature from artifice. Can it be that some of the things people take for granted to be harmless, right and good, are in reality bad?

Not long ago, such a question would have been met with scorn. But doubt has shattered ancient assumptions. Fat babies, once believed to be the healthiest of babies, are now known to be more likely to die than thin ones. If one chooses the largest, showiest vegetables on a stall, one is all the more likely to be buying the products of overfertilized soils, now known to be the source of the cancer-inducing nitrosamides, as well as a lashing of some insidious pesticide.

For all its sensational discoveries, science has turned out to be an unreliable guide. Indeed, it is largely responsible for a planetary outrage of nature, now threatening human survival. This crisis of malpractice and of misunderstanding the meaning of nature has been so well advertised, that no one should be able to delude himself today that things are not really as bad as they seem, that they will turn out to be all right in the end.

The sense of betrayal, of hopelessness, felt by many, especially the young, is understandable, for if the human being is without reliable guidance, in the artificial conditions of industrial civilization, disaster is certain. Having abandoned the gods, and now discovered the unreliability of reason and science, what hope remains? This is an attempt to show that the strongest hope of all, neglected by a matter-of-fact culture, is to be found in the human sensitivities—to beauty and purity in particular. It will be seen to be applicable to life's most important biological activity—eating.

In order to substantiate this claim, it will be necessary to begin by defining what is meant by the human sensitivities. To understand the meaning of beauty, so out of tune in a world dominated by materialistic values, will be to provide a basis for an approach to living radically different from the one taken by most people.

The value of science is not denied. The orderliness of nature discovered by science is one of the greatest achievements of the human spirit. But the way this evidence is used depends on some sustaining background of thought and belief. The mechanistic, materialistic ideal of present day science is by no means the only one possible. That it is inadequate, is indicated by the considerable amount of evidence which refuses to fit into the official picture of nature, and which is accordingly neglected.

The vision of nature which sustains this book is one of a Creation seeking wholeness, harmony, and beauty, and culminating in a creature able to appreciate these qualities, and to express them, and in so doing, to experience a sense of joyful participation in the Creation. There is ample evidence for such a vision, in the harmonies of atomic order as in the progressive achievement of beauty in the course of evolution.

In attempting to account for the human needs in food in calories and proteins, in minerals and vitamins alone, these other essential contributions which food can make to the human estate have been neglected. It is hoped that the subject will confirm that a reliance on the human sensitivities provides a valid and invigorating guidance to the way of life able to ensure harmony with nature, wholeness and health.

8

2. In Praise of Beauty

The way in which human beings appreciate beauty, and express it in their lives, and in their arts, depends on the prevailing social conditions. In harsh, cruel and heartless times, beauty goes out of living. The appeal of a Negro mask, of a medieval gargoyle, as of many modern pieces of sculpture, has more to do with excitement, sexiness, awe, with magic and other strange enticements than with beauty. In extreme conditions, the human mind becomes so anguished that it acquires a taste for the hideous and macabre, as in the cherished skull museums of head-hunters. Beauty in fact requires sufficiently humanizing, benevolent conditions.

With the Industrial Revolution, the beauty-loving Renaissance was superseded by a desecration of nature, and the rising of a man-made environment too often hideous and disorderly. The word beauty has gone out of fashion even among the lovers of art. It is sadly true that the periods of history benevolent enough for beauty to reign have been few.

Many have seen in this apparently natural lack of beauty the evidence that the appreciation of beauty, order and harmony is a cultural acquisition and not a genetic endowment. Those who have favoured a hard, aggressive view of man have seen in the preoccupation with beauty the evidence of decadence. Yet there is sufficient anthropological evidence that the more benign primitives, living in the more benevolent environments, have a natural appreciation of beauty, and express it in everything they touch, in every gesture, movement and ritual. In these conditions such a sensitivity to beauty goes hand in hand with an over-all compassionate disposition absent among the more harassed primitives, and among the civilized.

But the strongest indication that the beautiful is as indispensable a human feature as brain or upright posture, is the extraordinarily intense emotionalism associated with it, and the abundance of pleasure it can afford. That the appreciation of beauty is part of the humanizing process is shown by the humanizing effect such an appreciation has on human behaviour and predisposition in general. As the evolutionists would say, it has survival value.

The opposite of beauty is ugliness, synonymous with the bestial, with the mean, selfish and sordid, the disgusting and the sickly, all hostile to the human condition. Had the earliest humans not sensed the difference between ugliness and beauty, humanization would have come to an end. The distinction between beauty and ugliness runs close to the distinction between good and evil, between order and disorder. An evolving, learning brain requires a prolonged familial and social nature, which in turn was only possible in an orderly and harmonious social setting.

The capacity for love is leagued with a sensitivity to beauty. Many psychologists have observed that love is the guarantee of the mind's stability and wholeness, and that love-failure, in hatred, violence and viciousness, is the agent of the mind's disintegration. The appreciation of beauty, like love, can be defined as a condition of wholeness, and a sensitivity to that quality in others and in nature, providing the utmost degree of mental balance, of joy and a sense of meaningfulness in living. Whole food, fit for humans can but be beautiful food.

3. Beauty Pursued

So important has beauty been in human evolution, that one can expect the human being to be designed to find beauty in every possible thing, in every possible way. Nothing would be undertaken unless it had an aesthetic element to it. Such a beatific condition can still be observed among the few simple peoples left. In the islands of the Pacific, among the native tribes of Central America, people are bedecked with flowers, eating and love-making take place in flowered boweries, every object is made attractive and colourful, and the naked body variously adorned. The human body is felt rightly to be the object of supreme beauty, which accounts for the common nakedness.

One can learn much from the body's beauty, as the great masters of European painting realized. All beauty is there incarnate. The limbs are felt to be ideally proportioned, the smoothness of the skin inviting touch and caress, the eyes particularly enticing. The disappearance of body hair in the course of humanization has not only been due to the presumably temperate conditions in which human evolution occurred, but, of much greater importance, represents the removal of animal associations. What is left of the hair, around the head and, in the man, around the face, is evidently a haloing and an adornment, with an emotional effect the very opposite of animal. The only part of the body where the hair has not been aesthetized, and remains animal in its appeal, is around the genitalia. In a creature depending on social and familial harmony for survival, a primary interest in the genitalia would have been self-defeating. Consequently, the genitalia, and the hair associated with them, were left uncouth and unattractive, with the obvious intention of detracting attention from these parts. In a creature sensitized to beauty, this would be as good a way as one could find of ensuring that human relationships were not primarily sexual. All those primitives who live in an essentially naked condition, help nature by covering over the genitalia. A complete nudism, as much as clothing, is an expression of the aesthetic impoverishment of civilization; both are unnatural.

The female breast is a part of the body made particularly beautiful, intended to serve as the focus of a love, erotic, compassionate and social, echoing the ancient mammalian lineage of mankind. Many of the great painters of the Renaissance were alive to this appeal, picturing the infant Jesus suckled with exposed breast by Mary. There is something profound in this, for the mammalian female was emotionalized long before the male in the selfless devotions of mother love. In an important sense, the woman is more profoundly human than the man. But the echo of the breast in the man is a reminder also of his mammalian kind. Threatened male gorillas will beat their breasts like the angered elders of the Bible. When men confronted one another in battle in a naked condition, slaughter was minimal, compassion the rule.

The human infant has been made beautiful in a particularly tender, appealing way. It is interesting to note that the young of all mammals share in this appeal. However ugly the adult may appear, their young are invariably felt to be appealing, beautiful. In this tender appeal, an important attribute of beauty is apparent—its denial of an opportunist, bestial sexuality. This is absolute in the case of the infant; only the sick and the depraved feel sexually drawn to the children. But it is also evident, on another scale, in the erotic appeals of the adult body, wherein caress, adoration and tenderness can transfigure what can otherwise be an animal encounter. It is in this sense that human sexuality becomes transformed from the essentially reflex activities of animals into a sexual love felt to be pure, noble and beautiful.

Beauty is incompatible with impurity, so much so that the demand for purity is threaded in all the human sensitivities, in the very structure and function of the brain and mind. In the visual arts, there is an awareness of the purity of line, of form, of colour essential to the expression of beauty. So potent is this transfiguring quality, that even lewd and revolting subjects can become transformed, raised to a higher level of appeal, through the materials and techniques of art. Mere sexuality acquires an elysian quality, an eroticism steeped in ecstasy. Hence the clash of pornography, which is never art, and the erotic, which can be high art. The current habit of labelling attractive, beautiful things as 'sexy' betrays a sad corruption of perception and feeling.

Unless beauty was inherent and abundant in nature, it is unlikely that it could ever have played a role in humanization. Although the industrially jaded eye can become blind to the beauty of nature, once the veil is lifted, it is everywhere apparent still. Minerals can be very beautiful, and as minerals must have appeared at the dawn of Creation, as the first matter cooled sufficiently, one can conclude that matter is inherently endowed with beauty. Today, one knows that the beautiful symmetry of crystals, their amazing geometric purity, is the echo of atomic order. Since all things large or small are dependent on this order, one can be confident that nature is basically aesthetically compatible, a reassuring conclusion. This confidence is confirmed by the fact that beauty is increasingly expressed as evolution progresses. The ugliness of the early insects gave way to the beauty of the butterfly, the gawky pterodactyl emancipated into the bird of paradise, and the monotonous swamps of the Carboniferous were succeeded by the spectral orgies of flowers in the Cretaceous.

Without such a long preparation, persistently bringing out the latent beauty in things and creatures, the eventual emergence of a creature sensitive to beauty would have been impossible. Beauty in human existence remains closely dependent on beauty in the environment, in all things featuring in human life, which explains why an ugly age loses the meaning of beauty. Let us ponder well upon this, for it touches upon our subject intimately. Bearing in mind that the Creation is a whole, the evolution of beauty in landscape, in flowers, in human beings, in art, and, as we shall see, in such an important activity as eating, makes for a vast and intricate ecology of the beautiful. Unless harmonious forms were in existence before the earliest human appeared, in the wonderful shapes of hills, of trees, of pebbles, of shells, it would not have been possible for the earliest men to make the beautiful tools which accompany their remains. Unless flowers and fruits were already there, to provide the external stimuli of colour, human eyes would have been incapable of evolving the exceptional human sensitivity to colour. Creative evolution must have something to work on.

One can go further in affirming, in contradiction to the depressing and bestial origins now popular, that the human genesis must have occurred in an environment in which beauty and harmony prevailed, conditions which are recalled in the world-wide myths of an earthly paradise.

If the essential human mark, the distinction from the other hominids and higher primates, is not so much anatomy, but the sensitivity to love and beauty, care and compassion, virtues required for a most exacting breeding co-operation needed by an evolving brain, then truly human creatures may go back several million years. They are then likely to have had smaller brains, but a large brain is not necessarily a mark of humanization. The perfection of the organs connected with the humanizing sensitivities—the eye's sensitivity to colour, the olfactory sense to the perfume of flowers, the musical propensities of the human voice, must have taken a long, long time to perfect. This is an important inference, for it suggests that the most distinctive and characteristic human features were laid down before the advent of the Ice Ages, when near paradisiacal conditions prevailed in

14

many parts of the world. The fossil hominid evidence so far gathered may have nothing to do with this ancient human line, referring rather to the deviant, ruthless and murderous experiments, doomed to failure, spurred into being by the dehumanizing conditions of the Ice Ages.

If the human genesis occurred in conditions of beauty, then it must follow that what is naturally beautiful is likely to be humanly compatible, what is ugly, incompatible. This provides an intuitive guidance, quite different from common sense and reason, which has the backing of the whole of nature, and indeed has the backing of science, although most scientists are clueless as to the relevance of beauty. Nonetheless, some leading mathematicians and physicists have found that their theories are all the more likely to be true and valid, the more beautiful and harmonious they happen to be.

This intuitive guidance should be applicable to all human problems. Human beings can exist in the most horrid and terrible conditions, but they are bound to be all the less effectively human for it. The great civilizations of the past endeavoured to respect nature's inspiring beauty when ever possible, and to bring beauty to all man-made things. Whatever the tensions and frustrations inevitable in the complexities of civilization, there was thus a corrective humanizing force. With the industrial age, and with the dominance of the mechanical and materialistic viewing of science, this wisdom has been smothered, in a world grown mean and ugly.

Granting the importance of beauty, it is impossible to believe that food felt to be ugly and revolting, no matter how widely eaten, can be natural human food. Indeed, one would expect that such an important function would be made especially beautiful and humanizing. Pleasantly tasting natural foods are attractive, beautiful foods. Alas, in no other field have human beings shown such subterfuge in making what is naturally repulsive pass as attractive. The tragedy of human feeding lies here.

4. Beauty and the Beast

An Arcadian vision of mankind clashes with reality. Although most people have their better moments, it is violence, cruelty and horror that have dominated human history, and, from all the available evidence, ruled the lives of the Hominids in the Palaeolithic. This fact has encouraged the belief that man originated in horror and depravity, and that it is only thanks to culture and eventual civilization that he has managed to rise above a despicable natural condition. It is difficult to look at this apparent contradiction calmly, for there can be no doubt that the realities of hard existence harden the heart and blunt the sensitivities. The Arcadian appears absurd and unacceptable. Often enough, the response is one of anger, of hatred for the mild and the beautiful, to be seen in the common wanton killing of birds and butterflies, the trampling of flowers and the desecration of nature.

Yet even if the moments of blessedness are few and far between, they indicate a formidable intensity of feeling when they do occur, so strong as to completely alter the course of life in many cases. Such power cannot have come into being without some biological advantage. To the extent that they reveal a quality to life which is different from the usual and ordinary, they should be seen to imply that there are aspects of the human being which differ from the common experience, and contradict what one usually assumes to be the human standard.

In the past, this dilemma was resolved by religious beliefs of one kind or another, fortified by myths and played upon by magic and superstition. Today, in the name of a liberation from this ancient condition, science has promoted the view of a meaningless universe, in which the human presence is a merely accidental one, a situation to which the human being appears quite unadaptable, no matter what the material rewards. The increase in the anger and violence of the age springs from deep archaic responses rebelling against this inhuman crisis. In such a situation, one must expect that people are not likely to be able to think clearly and impartially, that bias and prejudice, even on the part of science, are bound to be rife, that any attempt to frame a different picture of the meaning of being human will be arbitrarily ruled out.

The evidence of the breakdown of the thin rational crust of the human mind is everywhere, to the extent that it has become very difficult to define what one is to mean by a normal state of mind. The Arcadian view of man provides such a definition concisely—the mind being normal only when the humanizing predispositions predominate, ensuring a wholeness of function in which benevolence and beauty prime, ruling out all that is mean, selfish and inhuman and providing a sense of joy and meaningfulness in living.

In such a happy state, the sub-human stages which the mind of every individual must carry, are silent. But they are easily aroused by any condition which wars against the forces of humanization. Lovelessness, a violent, mean, drab existence in an ugly hostile world, become the historical and well-nigh universal causes of an incipient mental pathology, the clash between beauty and the aroused beast, expressed in world-wide myths. As the sub-human minds are aroused, so the sub-human and anti-human passions that go with them come to take over human lives.

The mind is not without resources of defence against this disturbing onslaught. The humanizing predispositions are intensified, and given a social boosting, a process Freud described as the influence of the super-ego. But because the pressures can never be completely deviated by an imposed

morality and social censure, by religious and other sublim-
ating agencies, all societies have provided for periodical
venting of accumulated pressures, indispensable for their
survival with some degree of integration and order, from
competitive gambits and games, to warfare. It is not difficult
to find numerous examples in the competitive structures of
daily existence. The sadism, lust, and violence in entertainment are such outlets.

These existentially aroused subhuman aspects of the mind,
purulently affecting human behaviour, refer to a time
anteceding the human genesis. They know nothing of beauty,
of order, of harmony, of selflessness and love. Like all animal
passions, they are instinctual, immediately demanding,
callous and blind. Beauty, goodness and purity become
obstacles to their venting.

Although a preoccupation with the mystical and the occult
is a normal human interest, an expression of man's defiance
of matter and time, the magical is clearly antihuman, in its
relish of the macabre, the sordid, and the ugly. While mystical experience is invariably associated with beauty, the
magical purposefully excludes beauty and obliges a relish
in the obscene and the excremental. Today, there is a discernible arousal of the magical mind. Indeed magic has
never been fully quenched by the rise of reason; many aspects
of so called civilized life reveal it. Eating habits are not
without their magical asides.

If the mark of the human is a need for the beautiful, and
if the magical shows itself by a relish for the hideous, it is
simple enough to pick out the features of the diet which
are magical—the bloody joint, the dripping steak, organs
like the kidney concerned with filth elimination, foul smell-
ing foods, the desecration of living things which the killing
and cooking of any animal entails. This magical relish can
go to extremes, which then acquire a gruesome twist, as in
the chewing of eyeballs and the gobbling of brains, the
sucking of marrow and the savouring of testicles.

The point is that once the magical mind is aroused, such

18

practices are felt to be exciting, strength giving, indispensable, and in fact become supported by a corrupted reason,
by science itself. Just as the politician uses his reason to
justify an atomic overkill, entailing the murder of millions,
so the nutritionist assures one that fried brains are a good
source of protein. This is the frailty of reason—its easy misuse
for inhuman ends by minds no longer sufficiently irradiated
by the humanizing resources.

There is a sinister ally to such humanly debasing habits.
Protein products foreign to the normal physiology of the
body provoke chaotic reactions when eaten. In a wild attempt
to allay the intruding substances, the body produces too
much of the allaying chemicals, an excess which has the
malicious result of demanding more, and ever more, of the
foreign substances. The essential abnormality of all animal
foods is shown by the habituation and craving they provoke,
a demand which can come to defy all sense and economy.

In this manner, eating habits which comply with the
secret desires of a disturbed mind are fortified by an insidious biochemistry.

Food habits also reflect the life-hatred which goes with a
hardening of the heart to a hardened existence, as in the
barely believable hideousness of the death-dealing industries
supporting every civilized table. This life-hatred, and the
hatred of nature which accompanies it, goes back to the onset
of the Ice Ages, which chased the earliest humans from their
earthly paradise. No longer guided by instinct, but by cortical
conditioning, human beings are able to adopt virtually any
ruse in order to survive, no matter how unbiological. But
the fact that humanization occurred in idyllic conditions,
left humans badly equipped for the periodical geological
and climatic cataclysms of earth history. While in all other
animals, instinct would insist that the normal habits were
reverted to as soon as conditions returned to normal, in the
case of man, cortical conditionings, revived in each succeed-
ing generation by social customs, tend to persist. Animal
foods, and the vast machinery of suffering their eating entails,

have become one of the most entrenched of social customs, defended by science as natural and beneficial, and ardently insisted upon by the public.

Admittedly, attempts are made to give such horrible habits a veneer of aesthetic appeal. Cooking of animal foods removes the reek of raw flesh, and sauces help to smother the sheer animality of the ingredients. Here and there, vegetables, fruits and even flowers come into the decoration of some recipe as if to humanize the offence, sometimes ludicrously, as the ears of roast pork stuffed with flowers. But the underlying ugliness is scarcely covered, as most children show in their initial protests.

One is entitled to enquire how it is that science, which claims to operate on impartial reasoning, has failed to point out the unbiological and irrational features in such patently inhuman habits. The environmental crisis is proof enough that science is no impartial observer to the follies of an age, of a culture, and indeed serves them faithfully. Most scientists, and science as a whole, show the same spirit of aggressiveness and inconsideration regarding nature which dominated Palaeolithic existence.

The science of nutrition shows this insensitivity more than most. While physics and astronomy tend to attract the philosophers, nutrition seems to entice the extroverts, with an aversion to more profound thinking, in league with the disinclination to food fussiness shared by the common man. The fact is that nutritional science arose in a time when the industrial revolution had so disorganized an ancient way of life as to make poverty and undernutrition the rule among the masses, and the European influence in many parts of the world had sabotaged long-tried food habits and let loose widespread starvation. Nutrition has accordingly been haunted by insufficiency, and has been preoccupied with ensuring quantity. It is only quite recently that excess has been seen as a danger as much as deficiency.

But the philosophy of biology has also been guilty of failing to provide such a subsidiary science as nutrition with proper

20

guidance. Vieing to comply with the mechanical ideals, most biologists have been singularly blind to the most explicit characteristic of life, its functional integration and wholeness, in terms of which alone a living organism can be normal. As a result, biological thinking has largely missed the meaning of normality, and commonly mistaken the average for the normal. According to this crude way of thinking, since most people are in some way sick, sickness must be the normal human condition, and since most people like eating meat, meat eating is normal. Nutrition, in line with the thinking and feeling of the age, has been crude and permissive, backing the common greeds and perversions of taste with the hollow voice of authority.

As a result, bad, inhuman food habits, inherited from the Ice Ages, have been made more widespread and acceptable than they might otherwise have been, for in the past, the peasantries, whenever circumstances permitted, adopted dietary habits much closer to the human norm than usually prevails among the scientifically guided civilized. Under the banner of emancipation, nutritional science has in fact helped to make available to the masses the greeds and perversions once the preserve of the privileged classes.

Nature is not mocked. The price paid for this conspiracy is colossal. Given sufficient time, science may well become wiser and a better guide. In the past decades, its crudities have given way to a greater degree of sensitivity, of humility when faced with the complexities of living phenomena. But there is in all probability not enough time. In hatred and ugliness, man will have exterminated his own kind long before. It has become a desperate survival necessity to find an alternative meaning to being human, a change which is likely to demand a revolution in all human aspects and activities, most of all, in that most important of functions, eating.

5. Flowers, Fruits and Brain Cells

Until the Cretaceous period, the Age of Chalk, which began 136 million years ago and lasted 71 million years, there was little colour in the world, apart from the mostly hidden colour of minerals, the greens of chlorophyll, and the blues of sky and water. Then a remarkable event occurred. The leaves of certain plants became modified, in the incredibly rapid time of a few million years, into sepals and petals, which became filled with the brightest of pigments, providing thousands of different hues. At the same time, insects, which had been fearsome, ugly if not revolting creatures until then, also became resplendent in colour. As if not to be left out, the ungainly reptiles managed to sire some of the most exquisite of coloured creatures, the tropical tree lizards, and tropical fish became iridescent living jewels. Clearly, nature at that time had moved into an orgy of artistic expression.

As already suggested, the lavish presence of flowers in the environment of human genesis was indispensable for the evolution of the human colour sense. Botanists believe the origin of flowers occurred somewhere in Southern Asia, judging from the diversity of floral species still surviving there, as well as of some of the more primitive kinds. It is from there that flowers have spread all over the world, some regions and continents being more favoured than others. Another momentous event occurred in the Cretaceous which greatly influenced this distribution, and may have played a hand in the creation of the mammals, for this manmaking line also arose in the Cretaceous.

Prior to the Cretaceous, the continents had been amassed together around Africa; they then began drifting apart. Asia and the Americas moved the furthest away. The flowers spread easily all over EuroAsia, except in those regions then covered by ocean—regions now occupied by immense deserts and high mountains, the Himalayas. The flowers also occupied the Americas, by a landbridge with Asia which persisted into human times. Africa, however, possessed a considerable obstacle to the spread of flowers—an ocean, which is now the Sahara, and the impenetrable tropical forest-belt stretching right across the continent. As a result, Africa is a continent poor in floral species, except for the north, where flowers have crept in from the near East, and in the extreme south, where flowers may have travelled by a landbridge with Asia over what is now only a scattering of islands across the Indian Ocean.

The fact that EuroAsia is richer in flower species than Africa would indicate that humanization is more likely to have occurred somewhere in Asia, as was once believed, rather than in Africa, now the most favoured site, in view of the large number of hominid remains found there. But as anthropologists agree, this may be fortuitous; abundant remains may yet be found in Asia, or possibly once abundant remains have been subsequently effaced by geological events, which have been particularly intense in Asia, with the rising of the Himalayas, still rising when the earliest men were on the scene. This inference is further supported by the fact that the low lying fruits, like the apple family, which presumably formed the essential part of the food of the ground living pre-human apes, are virtually uniquely the product of Asia. In other words, the numerous fossil hominids of Africa may be no more than hominid experiments, with little or nothing to do with the true human line. This would be just as well, for the African hominids were a blood-thirsty, cannibalistic lot.

That fruits are the favourite foods of the higher Primates is explained by the fact that fruits offer one of the most concentrated supplies of energy in nature, owing to their high content of sugar. For animals with relatively large brains and complex social patterns, such a concentrated food enables much time to be spent in developing these characteristics, in the continual games and other social frolics so typical of these animals. Long browsing and searching would have barred social evolution. As a prelude to the evolution of man, fruits had an exceptional advantage—they are among the most beautiful and harmonious objects in nature.

A consequence of a largely fruitarian diet resulted in digestive changes, in the chimpanzee and in man, which had unexpected subsequent results. The concentrated energy of fruit sugars enabled a considerable reduction in the size and length of the alimentary tract in these two primates, compared with the bulky digestive organs of the gorilla, for instance, a primate living largely on tough leaves. It is this reduction which enabled man, and to a lesser extent, the chimpanzee, to take to eating animal foods when their natural diet fails.

The lengthy alimentary tract of the bulky plant eaters is quite incongenial to such a mixed diet, for the very opposite conditions are needed for the digestion of proteins or of plant fibres. The one has to be absorbed rapidly, and eliminated rapidly, before putrefactive poisons have time to accumulate, while the latter needs time for the nutrients to be digested out of the fibrous matrix. But this does not imply that man or chimpanzee is well adapted to have such a mixed diet, for a preponderance of proteins, which a mixed diet involves, required a revolution in metabolism as well. The metabolic end products of protein, like the putrefactive products formed in the gut by bacteria, call for very special devices so as to enable their excretion in a harmless form. All carnivores possess such deamination devices. The primates are entirely deprived of them, so that any intake of nitrogenous substances over a relatively low level of a vegetarian dietary, puts a strain on the system. Uric acid and other end products of purine metabolism accumulate, causing increas-

24

ing havoc over the years in rheumatic joints and kidney strain.

That the level of protein intake at which deamination is optimally efficient is identical in man and chimpanzee to that of the other primates, should make it clear that the rare sallies of chimpanzees into flesh eating, and the common mixed diet of humans, are emergency measures. Since protein metabolism is the most difficult aspect of digestion, one must expect that a physiological tax has to be paid for defying its natural limits. This is an important question, for if the human being required the relatively large amounts of protein recommended by nutritionists—1 gram per kilo body weight—then man would have had to be a 'mixed eater' from the start, and could not be the preponderantly fruit-arian creature suggested in this book. Since protein balance studies confirm that humans, like the other primates, need no more than about a third of this amount, one can only conclude that the standards recommended are wrong.

Because proteins are unquestionably important, nutritionists have thought it wise to set their standards according to the so called 'best fed nations', those peoples in fact who in all probability consume far more food altogether than they need. Nutritionists, doing field surveys in the tropics, have been surprised to find people living on amounts of protein much lower than they had been led to believe were indispensable, and living well and healthily. Although the writer found many other signs of malnutrition in the course of such a survey, he found no protein deficiency, except in places where malaria was rife. In fact, the lurid picture of protein deficiency in textbooks on the subject only occur in exceptional conditions of general famine following wars and other catastrophes.

The beauty of fruits, their sweetness and exquisite flavours, —how different those different varieties of apple, of pear, of peaches can taste!—are the ideal food for a beauty-loving animal. The conditions in the Cretaceous which brought colour to the world in flowers, so preparing the way for the evolution of the human colour sense, also brought into being the fruits on which the highest of creatures, the most noble, beautiful and pure, would in time come to feast. The human being is best designed as a picker of fruits, not a climber of tall trees, so that only low growing fruit trees would meet his needs. It is just these fruits that abound, and abound still, in the EuroAsian landmass—particularly the apple family, so close to the rose, and also peaches, cherries, plums, apricots, grapes and a multitude of berries. The high growing fruit of tropical jungles could have fed only a few acrobats.

The apple features as the miraculously healing fruit in the folklores of many of the peoples of EuroAsia. In many of their languages, apple is synonymous with fruit. The myth of Adam and Eve recounts the drama of the Fall, the chasing from the earthly paradise, no doubt by the Ice Ages, and the human corruption which ensued. In offering the apple, Eve was symbolically reminding the man that lust could only be pursued at the loss of a natural purity, of wholeness. In eating the apple, Adam destroyed the symbol of human purity, and the human race began its long stumble into pain and misery. In an engraving by Dürer, it is the snake, phallic symbol of lust, which eats the apple.

The human need for very large amounts of daily fruit is borne out by the relative enormous amounts of vitamin C needed for optimal health and general well-being. The primates are exceptional in their needs for this vitamin, for almost all other animals, including pure vegetarians like the rabbit make their own requirements of it. Although the human being, like the other primates, can make do with smaller amounts of vitamin C in their foods, they are less fit for it, more prone to infections, listless and unhappy. The common cold is common because commonly people do not eat enough fruits. The official recommendations, in all other respects probably excessive, appear to have underestimated the needs of vitamin C, judging from the ever increasing list of diseases in which an inadequacy of this vitamin is involved. The reason for this underestimating is simple. Not

26

believing man to be basically fruitarian, they have ignored the hints that have come up over the past years for much larger needs of vitamin C, for such amounts could only be met by living largely on fruits.

The primates are lured to fruits by their colour, by their pleasant smell and feel, and particularly, by their sweet taste. Many animals have something of a sweet tooth, but nowhere as marked as that of human beings. In a natural world, to eat sweet things is to eat vitamin C. The child's craving for sweets is in reality a craving for fruits, which shows up the iniquity of confectionery, the biggest nutritional deception ever devised and responsible for much pain and misery. Besides sweetness, the acidity of fruits is also an enticement to eating them. Not only do such acids clean the mouth without dissolving the enamel of the teeth, squeezing the salivary glands and providing the right milieu in the digestive tract, but there is evidence that in their metabolism, they have a tonic effect on the body as a whole.

This insistence on fruits on the part of nature must have some special significance to humanization. The cortex of the brain alone has some six thousand million cells, each cell intertwined in a profusion of interconnections. This inconceivably complicated structure can only function if a perfect co-ordination prevails. A few molecules of some undesirable substance sends the whole mechanism out of gear. Anything less than a perfect co-ordination is insanity. It stands to reason that in evolving such a fantastic organ, natural selection would have picked on a way of life, including a way of feeding especially, which could have best ensured this cerebral equilibrium.

The brain's need of vitamin C is higher than any other tissues. The brain functions on sugar, which fruits ideally supply. But it is the fact that a preponderantly fruitarian diet necessarily means a low protein diet which is probably the fruits' particular advantage in brain evolution, for even in those animals long adapted to a high protein diet, the carnivores, the tissue wear-and-tear, and the cumulative

27

damage by the products of protein metabolism, are not completely overcome. The carnivores are short-lived, and quick-growing, the opposite conditions for evolving a large, long-learning brain.

Sharing the mechanistic bias of biology, nutritionists have popularized the subject of protein by stressing the simplicity whereby the body picks its own requirements of amino acids from the welter of proteins eaten, implying that it does not matter what the source of protein happens to be as long as all the amino acids are provided in abundance; that eating other animals is the best way of meeting this seems evident to such a mentality. But in the last decade, the barely believable complexity of protein chemistry has become apparent. There are a host of nitrogenous substances accompanying proteins which tag on to amino acid digestion and reassembly, thereby becoming a part of the body's chemistry. Only very minute amounts of such substances are involved, but their effects can be out of all proportion to their amounts. They can in fact act as drugs and hormones, and impinge upon those all-controlling submicroscopic wonders, the genes.

Because of the far greater complexity of the proteins in animals than in plants, such accessory nitrogenous substances are much more abundant in animal foods than in plant foods. In fact, they barely occur at all in fruits, while present to some extent in a few foods of vegetable origin, such as yeast and chocolate. It has recently been discovered that vitamin C helps in the metabolism and removal of these substances from the tissues, so that the importance of vitamin C in brain function is understood.

The pieces begin to fit in a most interesting way, for not only would fruits offer a minimum of potentially disturbing products of protein metabolism, but they would ensure that the brain is protected from the minor amounts that must arise on the most perfect diet. Since vitamin C cannot be stored in the tissues, nothing less than a daily abundance of fruits will meet the needs of a brain-evolving creature such as man. In fact, nature made no attempt to store the vitamin, as it made none to manufacture the vitamin in the human body, in order to make quite sure that human beings would gorge on fruits daily. Combined with the already mentioned advantage of providing a concentrated source of energy, with a minimum bulk, this makes fruits the essential condition of humanization. Had the earth not evolved flowers and fruits in that breath-taking splendour of the Cretaceous, humanization could not have taken place some one hundred and fifty million years later.

Because science has done nothing to encourage one to sense the unity of nature, such a feat of prevision seems incredible. But if nature is a whole, then it must follow that earlier stages prepare for the later ones, as in a living organism. One can conclude, with hope revived, that these many thousands of millions of years of evolution from stardust to mammals, had a definite developmental end in view—us. No doubt the cosmologists are right in assuming that life evolves into being in endless planets. But one can be reasonably assured that unless such planets bring forth flowers and fruits, among many other requirements, humanization would not be possible, and so a mind, able to sense the beauty and harmony of Creation, would be ruled out.

6. The Life-Giving Seeds

So important have fruits been to body and mind, that the quality and quantity of other nutritional essentials in an optional human diet are likely to be determined by the manner in which they fit into this fruitarian scheme. This has been hinted to be the case with protein.

It is a well-known principle that deficiencies in one part of a plant are made up in another. In the case of fruits, the deficiencies of the soft, sugar-soaked part are compensated for in the seeds. While the pulp of fruits contains very little protein, the seeds contain between 8 and 22 per cent. The nut is of course a fruit seed, the almond being the seed of a beautiful member of the apple family. Seeds and nuts also compensate for mineral and vitamin deficiencies of fruits. For instance, the pulp and the juice have very little of the B vitamins, and calcium, while seeds and nuts are rich in these essentials. In the fruit as a whole therefore, nature has offered a well balanced food.

Another example of such complementation is that between seeds and nuts, on the one hand, and leaves and shoots on the other. While many seeds and nuts have not much lysine, and methionine, amino acids indispensable for the manufacture of protein in the body, green growing leaves are full of them. Thus cereals by themselves, or with fruits, may be inadequate, but with green shoots they provide all the amino acids required, an example which insists that requirements be considered as a whole, as one should all things. Separate analyses are useful and interesting, but one should always sense their part in a thoroughly integrated scheme of nature; nothing properly exists in isolation.

Most fruits have diminutive seeds, and nuts are not over-abundant. The primates are communal animals, and a more plentiful supplement was indispensable. While some primates, like the gorilla, specialized in leaves, the human line took to the grasses, which produce seeds in abundance. Together with tender shoots, their ideal complement, the grasses, ancestors of the cereals, were most probably the in-ducement to living on the ground. As grasses are not to be found in the tropical forests, the home of the other higher primates, one must suppose that the human line, like the chimpanzee, had become ground-living under quite different conditions.

In the Miocene, some sixty million years ago, the Himalayas had barely begun their stupendous rise from the bed of a gigantic ocean once stretching from the Atlantic to the Pacific. The rising land must have produced many lakes —the Black Sea, the Caspian and the Mediterranean are such survivors—and gently sloping, well-watered valleys in which flowers prospered. Conditions possibly not very different persist to this day in the flower- and fruit-filled valleys south of the Central Asian Plateau. Conditions were also ideal for the grasses. In the more temperate regions, these were relatively short growing, enabling especially adapted trees—the typical temperate tree flora and especially the fruit trees, which are well suited to a grassy environment —to grow interspersed with grass, producing orchard- and park-like conditions.

The Miocene saw the rise of that great family of grass eaters, the herbivora. Their virtual defencelessness indicates that these were also benevolent times, when beasts of prey were few. These are better adapted to the jungles of the tropics, and the tall grasses of the tropical savannas. The carnivora cannot persist long in a chase—the nature of their diet hinders long sustained effort—so that they must surprise their prey and kill quickly and surely, conditions not met in

31

the short grass lands of the semi-tropical and temperate regions.

In all probability, it is these conditions which persisted into the Pliocene, which lured the hominid ancestors to become ground-living, thus isolating themselves from the other primates which followed the retreating tropical vegetation as the world climate became colder as the Miocene passed into the Pliocene. The popular notion that our ancestors took to the ground in order to prey on game is nonsensical. Man is not equipped as a natural hunter; in every hunting community, he has to learn the skills of hunting the hard way. That human beings have lived as intermittent hunters since the onset of the Ice Ages does not alter the fact that their bodies remain totally unadapted to this way of life. Man's gait and posture, the remarkable co-ordination of hand and eye, the entire digestive and metabolic equipment, point to a native plant food-gatherer, an activity calling for communal co-operation and participation which is at the heart of socializing drives.

From the first therefore, the abundant seeds of the grasses probably formed an intrinsic part of man's diet. In many parts of the world to this day, handfuls of grass seeds can be easily collected by sieving the spathes through the fingers. Such seeds have the further advantage that they will keep; they can be eaten raw, or ground into flour and made into porridge, pancakes, biscuits, chappatis and the endless varieties of flour usage found all over the world. With the ending of the Ice Ages some ten thousand years ago, it was inevitable that mankind should set about selecting the most congenial of the grasses, so bringing into being the cereals, closer to the nuts in size, and virtually identical in composition.

It is this ideal human diet of fruits, shoots and seeds which enabled the evolution of society, for its concentration made much time available for social activities. In bringing about a reduction in the length and size of the alimentary tract, it enabled man also to eat other foods, far from his ideal, in order to survive during the Ice Ages. In a mind-bearing creature, such a departure from the ideal is likely to have had the most disturbing effects on the mind. In the next chapter, the way in which this transgression of natural law has affected the human mind will be traced.

7. The Sources of Evil

It was earlier mentioned that human needs for protein are lower than is usually stated, and that animal foods not only provide an excess of protein, but introduce into the body economy unnatural nitrogenous substances. It is a biological law that an animal can only deal efficiently with substances to which it has become adapted in the course of its long evolution. Changes in size and shape can be brought about in a few generations, but functional changes require much more time. Recent estimates of the time necessary for evolving quite different metabolic and enzymatic lines, such as would be incurred in a radical change of diet, runs into many millions of years. In every function studied, man remains identical to the higher primates, to the chimpanzee, the gorilla and the gibbon in particular, which means that the nearly universal 'mixed' type of human feeding is an abnormality and is bound to cause some sort of functional trouble. The possible consequences to the body have been pointed out from time to time by medical men and other scientists, but most people have considered the risks worth taking, if indeed they have been willing to accept the evidence of bodily damage at all. It is only recently that the effect on the mind has become more apparent. The price that has to be paid for such widescale dietary transgression seems truly enormous.

As far back as 1931, Quastel and Wheatley had indicated that certain products of protein digestion, especially those resulting from bacterial decomposition, possessed properties analogous to the most potent mind-affecting drugs such as mescalin, which might play a role in mental disturbances. At the time, this information was felt to be awkward, if not preposterous, possibly because it was felt unlikely that such an important item of food could be incriminated in mental disorder. Whatever the reason, it is only some forty years later that the problem was reopened, when the role of the monoamines in brain functioning was discovered. Ketz distinguishes between the biogenic amines, manufactured by the brain tissues, responsible for normal mental states, and a wide range of slightly altered monoamines which could be responsible for more unusual states, like mystical ecstasy, hallucinations and 'high' dreams. Between normality and psychosis, one might find a graduation of subtle alteration of the monoamine molecules.

Since mescalin was isolated in 1943, the biochemical connection of the more elusive aspects of human experience, in love, in the arts, in mystical and other states, has been apparent. Evidently, nature has made use of drug-like substances produced by the brain itself, such as reserpine. This does not imply that the mind 'is nothing but a chemical brew', but it does indicate that even the most elusive mental functions, such as the humanizing sensitivities, have a biological basis, an indication which should be obvious enough if the universe is a consistent enterprise. Although engendered by brain cells, there is every indication that mental experience in itself is not a part of the physical and chemical order. But whatever the nature of the mind, it is undoubtedly very much affected by biochemical events. There is a definite pharmacology of the soul.

The monoamines are products of protein metabolism, a fact which makes the proteins as important to the mind as to the body. The finer aspects of protein metabolism are only now beginning to be unravelled. For too long it has been crudely assumed that brain and body can manufacture their protein needs from any kind of food protein, so long as the chemical building blocks are supplied. Very slight changes in molecular structure, barely detectable by the chemist, can have profound effects on living functions, particularly in

35

such a precariously balanced one as the brain, with its billions upon billions of cells and interconnections. Ketz has suggested the possibility 'that the different amines give some characteristics to the newly synthetized proteins, imparting a "colour code" of affective qualities as it is being formed'. Very slight shifts from the normal might have enormous affective, emotional, behavioural consequences.

For every so called 'normal' protein that features in nutrition, there may be millions of such minor abnormal molecular variations. Although the body does possess an outstanding ability to select the protein ingredients it requires, this ability is only likely to refer to the ingredients which form part of the normal nutritional pattern, a pattern minutely and exactingly set by evolution. The possibility already referred to, of a wide confusion regarding the 'normal' in human nutrition, makes it possible that the human mind is exposed to protein products which are in various ways abnormal, with possibly momentous effects on brain function.

The abnormal amines could be both manufactured in the body during the metabolism of abnormal proteins, as well as by bacterial action on protein wastes in the alimentary tract, especially in the colon, on the nitrogenous products which have resisted absorption, usual in a 'mixed' diet. It is here that one can make a clear distinction between foods of animal origin, and of plant derivation. Besides the large amounts of proteins in animal foods, there are a host of substances related to the amines, the purines and the pyramidines, and those released by putrefactive changes. These form what analysts term the extractives, consisting of the more easily hydrolyzable and soluble protein products, and therefore all the more easily absorbed. These are completely absent in fruits and many vegetables, and only present in minor amounts in seeds and nuts. However, some plant foods do contain significant amounts also, as does cocoa, yeast extract, and many pulses.

On a diet of fruit and vegetables, low in protein, a fermentative bacterial flora prevails, which is biochemically the opposite of putrefaction, a living process in which yeasts are active, producing B vitamins and other substances useful to the body. Putrefaction is rightly associated with death. On a 'mixed' diet, not only is protein usually in excess, but the vegetable fibres present hinder the digestion of protein, providing more wastes for the putrefactive bacteria in the colon. One must conclude that the diet of most humans, the world over, is particularly favourable for the production and absorption of abnormal amines.

The normal monoamines would be presumably concerned in initiating the humanizing predispositions, the aspirations to goodness and harmonious social relationships, to love, compassion and co-operation, and the joys and ecstasies that go with their fulfilment. The more elusive, yet important pursuits of purity, of the mystical and spiritual, are connected. The abnormal amines, on the other hand, are disruptive rather than integrating, more likely to excite the lower, prehuman aspect of mind, normally quiescent but easily aroused, accounting for the mischief and the insensitivity in the human midst, and, when more severe, for the violence and hatred, the horrors and bestialities of existence.

To find such a biochemical basis to evil, in world-wide aberrations of diet, must appear as the over simplification of an immensely complex problem. Certainly no two individuals are likely to react in the same way to the same abnormalizing conditions, and some people will be better equipped than others to resist the inhuman tendencies, as some societies have been more active than others in encouraging an acceptable level of human behaviour. But statistically, over sufficient time, abnormal effects on the mind will push behaviour towards the inhuman and bestial. It is not the rarer outburst of loving, the sudden craving for beauty and purity, that count so much as the steady loading of thought, desire and action in directions which are subtly not properly human, for ever waiting for the periodical occasions for more terrible venting, in the tragedies of individual existence as in the recurring crises of human history.

8. Love, Lust and Aggression

The destructive anger and hatred of human beings serves no biological purpose; on the contrary, they are a threat to human survival. Although primates, and humans, are not territorial animals, in the sense that the carnivores are territorial, they do resent encroachment into their habitats. Gorillas can get very angry and ferocious. It is evident therefore that the capacity for anger has been purposefully retained in the evolution of the primates, to meet threat and challenge, even if their usual and normal patterns of existence are peaceful. As humans became hunters with the Ice Ages, they did in fact acquire some of the territorial predispositions of carnivores and hunting animals. This is understandable, for game is scarce at the best of times, a given area only being able to provide a tenth or less of game compared to vegetable foods. With this cortically involved territorialism, there has arisen a capacity for exercising anger, violence and ruthlessness. But this is not natural; it is purely existential.

If the usual is confused for the normal, it is impossible to make sense of the historical, and prehistorical, facts of man's extreme and unbiological aggressiveness. Attempts to find reasons and advantages for it, are fanciful. While aggressiveness as a normal pattern of life in many animals is clearly biologically advantageous, attempts to transpose such advantages to the human genesis entails an ignorance of the most pertinent human features, those which have been absolutely essential for the very special type of social organi-

38

zation characteristic of humans as opposed to the groupings found among other animals.

The fact is that most people have at one time or another known the meaning of love, if not fully in the reality of their lives, then at least in longing and in dreaming. Love is then seen to be a condition of joy nearing ecstasy, a desire to give oneself for others, a longing for the pure and the beautiful, the righteous and noble, so powerful as to completely transfigure the meaning of existence. In such moments, there is no possibility of meanness and selfishness, of brutality and cruelty. Clearly, such a humanizing predisposition, innate and biologically implanted, affecting all thought and behaviour, has been absolutely indispensable for the familial and social structure required by an evolving and a developing brain. In the fact of such requirements, any contrary suppositions can but amount to faulty and injurious myth-making. Since most people like to find support for what they happen to be, rather than for what they should be, such spurious myth-making, from which scientists themselves are not entirely absolved, are very popular.

The intensity of love's ecstasy, proving its biological implantation, is evidently designed to be kindled in an atmosphere of sexual love, the longing for another, calling for tenderness and solicitation, care and adoration. In such a scheme, the human body and the human face have necessarily been decreed by natural selection as the most beautiful things in the Creation, the ultimate objects of veneration. As sexual love is fulfilled, so comes a sense of profound meaningfulness in all things. Lovers have no doubt that life has meaning, that nature is sacred.

In such a state, mere carnality is transcended into a near divine rapture. Each touch becomes an act of adoration, each word and movement holy. There can be no blind demand for an animal stampede into the self-centred relief of immediate coitus. On the contrary, the love game overcomes time, and when coitus occurs, it is a sublime unitive rapture which thoroughly transcends flesh, place and time, in a 'high' whose

39

promise was whispered in the first encounters of loving.

This near divine transfiguration of the body, and thereby of the universe, in the 'high' of sexual love, is the complete opposite of the lewd and lustful, of the pornographic, purient interest in the body, in the sexual organs. The purity which it demands makes it the prerogative of youth, of young lovers. Although it carries an obvious ability to be shared with others, and with all things, it is the most naturally achieved in an enduring relationship with another. By definition, careless change and promiscuity are contrary to it.

The impulse to a wider sharing of love, originally awakened in sexual loving, takes also a sexless form of immense importance to a creature communally bonded by compassion rather than by instinct or advantage, in the love of family, of friends, of community, of nature. The natural tendency for love to spread out into non-sexual directions gives an indication of how sexual love itself should evolve among lovers, in a form the most congenial and useful to society. The pristine rapture of sexual love cannot last, and is not designed to do so, but rather to be progressively replaced by compassion, in the teaming of procreation, with interests shared, and, with advancing years, in a heightening social and spiritual involvement. Living, loving and ageing in such an atmosphere of evolving love, the human being is assured of a meaningful participation in the function and structure of family and society. And most other cultures have believed that human society symbolically reflects the underlying structure of Creation.

Such a definition of sexual love is so contradicted by the usual expression of sex in industrial societies, that it must appear as unreal and Utopian. Yet there is sufficient evidence that sexual love, rather than just sex, is the normal human pattern among simpler peoples, and among those few fortunate primities still surviving in the more benevolent habitats.

Having a top biological priority in humanization, one can

understand why the joys that attend the achievement of sexual love are the highest that can come to the human being, and why the failure to achieve love is accompanied by the most terrible misery and frustration, anger and hatred. Contrary to what the Freudians have claimed, guilt is a biologically implanted reprimand for sexual patterns which fail to comply with the needs of humanization. Since the precarious wholeness of the mind depends on the unifying forces of love, beauty and harmony, the failure to find love is punished by the most satanic of afflictions—an unwhole and disturbed mind.

The failure to achieve sexual love, more evident today than ever before, is to be seen in the breakup of the family, in selfish sexual opportunisms in the common uncaring for the young, and, as a result of this dehumanization of sexuality, in a soaring juvenile destructiveness and anger, in a general feeling of having been cheated of life's promise. Neglected, unloved, without the guidance which only genuine loving is entitled to provide, it is not surprising that the young have rebelled against the prurient standards set by callous and insensitive adults. The generation gap is the inevitable result of an older generation felt to be corrupt and lewd, the makers of a civilization which has become inhuman in its material-istic and opportunist preoccupations.

While it is true that many young subscribe in their own ways still to this civilization—imitation is after all the Simian way of learning—there are also those who have managed to recover something of the lost innocence, even if drugs have played their part in this recovery.

So demented is the sexual demand, so blind the pre-occupation with orgasmic relief, that the conclusion one is dealing with a pathological process appears irresistible. And there can be no doubt that the increase of social violence has gone hand in hand with an increase in this ferocious sexual pursuit, with an increase in uncaring and promiscuity. The association of sex with violence and human depravity is patent in entertainment, in pornography, as it is in group

41

outlets from gang behaviour to revolution and warfare.

For the past century, psychologists and sociologists have loudly proclaimed that guilt and repression are responsible for the frustrations and angers of the age. Sexual freedom has thus become the panacea for the ravaged modern soul. Many people have come to believe that the pursuit of the orgasm is a virtual duty, a recipe for healthfulness, in spite of the fact that the ability to contain the physical urge of sex, and find pleasure in so doing, must have been a necessity from the first steps in human evolution, without which an effective integration of the family and social group would have been quite impossible.

That frustration, the ally of anger and hatred, are the consequences of lust, of sexuality pursued without love, can be observed in the backwash of dissatisfaction that invariably follows the purely physical preoccupations of sexuality. This is particularly marked in the young; outbursts of violence, destructiveness, aggressiveness often follow periods of extreme licence among the youth gangs of large cities. One must therefore conclude that a socially disturbed mind is especially prone to any other disturbing influences that may impinge upon it, such as the abnormal mind-affecting amines in an abnormal diet.

The manner in which the higher aspects of the mind become sabotaged by the lower, is as yet little understood. Arthur Koestler, contemplating the overwhelming failure of human beings to be human, and the periodical insanity of human history, concludes that something must have gone wrong in the evolution of the brain. Others have speculated that viruses as yet undetected have infected parts of the brain controlling the sexual motivations. But there is a less far searching explanation in the virtually universal prevalence of the abnormal mind-affecting amines, which does not require such a bungling on the part of nature in the making of its highest work, the brain.

The 'lower emotions' such as fear, aggressiveness, and the blind copulatory drives, are known to originate in the limbic

42

system, a region a few centimetres thick which encapsulates the dilated end of the brain stem. The 'higher emotions' such as the humanizing sensibilities arise in a most complicated interplay between the cortex and the brain stem. It would seem that the role of the cortex is to transmute an ancient mammalian capacity for effective emotional experiences; some interchange between the limbic system and the most highly evolved humanizing aspects is accordingly natural and normal. But to conclude, as does P. D. Maclean, that this points to an evolutionary failure to wall off the primitive from the human, which would account for an ingrained paranoid streak, seems unjustified. The problem is functional, —the wrong 'colour' of the affective processes due to abnormal amine stimulation. The same faulty amines responsible for an overall disturbance of the mind and an arousal of its more primitive aspects, could account for the near demonic sexual drives of most humans, inducing a pattern of sexuality the very opposite of that intended by nature as the main agent in humanization.

This suggestion, that wrong foods can account for the pathology of sex, would find confirmation in the ancient belief that foods had aphrodisiac properties, an aphrodisiac being defined as a substance able to stimulate and titillate the lower sex emotions. Aphrodisiac foods are indeed those which have the highest amount of the extractives giving rise to the purines and amines.

9. Need or Greed

Besides the protein excesses involved in a so called 'mixed' dietary, the Industrial Revolution, entailing profound changes in the world production of food and in food habits, has led to an excessive eating of calorie foods, while some of the more minute requirements of the mind and body have gone in short supply, resulting in the malnutrition of abundance. This disturbing greed for the grosser items of foods, proteins and calories, has been achieved at the expense of the poorer, primary producers, making the greed of the so called best-fed nations a planetary affront.

Gluttony is never possible in nature, for food is never so plentiful as to permit a continual overeating. Occasional orgies may occur, the result of a lucky find, but they are inevitably interspersed by longer periods of scarcity. The only overfed animals are the pets of overfed people. The bodies of all animals are better adapted to scarcity than to abundance, which is what one would expect, given the geological and climatic restlessness of the earth. As food supplies become more scarce, reserves are mobilized, the body becomes more sparse, more active, and clutter vanishes. One finds people in the poorer parts of the world existing in apparent health, skinny but very active and smiling, on much less than the authorities consider should bring about starvation. While living on such low levels is to be deplored, it does show that the human body is remarkably well adapted to adversity, in fact thrives on it. Some degree of it, at least occasionally, may be indispensable for health, for the body seems to have become

44

adapted to profit from such periods in order to get rid of old stock, of accumulated wastes, the means also of resharpening the senses and the efficiency of functioning, taking in the slack and repairing damage.

The sense of well-being, of elation and purification which follows a period of abstinence from food shows that this is natural, biologically beneficial. Such benefits may not be immediately apparent in the chronically overfed or the diseased, for in them the respite from abuse is taken advantage of by the body for a massive, and often disturbing broom sweeping. But even then, persistence is rewarded by a remarkable quickening of all the faculties, by a sense of reawakening and rejuvenation and a simple joyfulness which most people have not known since childhood. Scents and colours, feelings and tastes long lost are magically revived, and simple pleasures, which seemed boring to the surfeited mind and body, return with a pristine intensity. The humanizing sensitivities are particularly revived, bringing about an awareness of harmony and beauty in things and creatures previously neglected.

It is remarkable to observe how the reactivity of the body as a whole is heightened. Long established chronic ailments may disappear overnight, and blights that have haunted and humiliated for years, itches and bodily odours, vanish as with a magician's wand. This is not surprising, for contrary to the usual assumption that even a temporary abstinence is dangerous, the body is designed for it and thoroughly enjoys it. The common supposition that even a skipped meal is a calamity boosts the common gluttony. It is not found among the simpler peasantries. Hard work and thrift ensure lithe bodies and alert minds into old age. There are still such examples surviving, peasants setting out for a long hard day's work with no more than a few dried figs or dates, a chunk of coarse bread dipped in olive oil, a garlic or two and an occasional piece of cheese. The Chinese peasants will perform feats of endurance and labour on what seems to the overfed European diminutive bowls of rice with scatterings of beans.

45

The scramble for food originated with the rise of the cities, for while the peasants could always eke some sustenance from their land in the worst of times, the cities often starved, as a consequence of plunder, famine, and pestilence. When good times came, city people stuffed themselves, so that over-eating became the mark of prosperity and privilege.

As privileged classes arose, ruling the cities and taking over the land, with power over supplies, gluttony became their habit, while the masses often knew hunger. The situation grew worse with the rise in power of the city states in the Middle Ages, and very much worse with the Industrial Revolution. Its initial impact brought such disorder that starvation often overtook the cities.

As a result of this background of general scarcity, the demand for food, and ever more food, was the pivot of all the movements of emancipation which began actively in the seventeenth century. This demand was eventually met by the agricultural revolution, the use of chemical fertilizers, the importation of foreign foods in exchange for industrial products and the refining of cereals, which enabled prolonged storage and easy transportation. Food production was thus geared to quantity rather than quality.

A century ago, every reasonable person would have praised the measures taken by the authorities and the industrialists, and blessed the scientists who were increasingly responsible for processed natural foodstuffs, increasing their size and yield, introducing preservation, colouring, conditioners and a soaring list of chemicals. But in a rising spiral of disaster, the arrogant interferences with nature have become apparent in the recent decades, in a planetary ecological collapse.

Excessive applications of chemical fertilizers, with insufficient or absent organic contributions, have led to a breakdown of some of the world's most fertile soils, calling for ever higher applications in a desperate attempt to keep up the yield, and ending in disasters like the American Dust Bowl. More recently it has been found that excess nitrate fertilizers are accumulated in food plants, and, when eaten, are converted to the highly cancerous nitrosamides. The over-spill of nitrates into rivers and lakes, encouraging the prolific growth of toxic blue-green algae, has sterilized many waters with once abundant fish life.

Mineral nitrates are manufactured into proteins by plants, the source of all animal protein. Too much nitrate abnormally stimulates plant growth, just as too much protein abnormally stimulates the growth-rate and size of animals. Superficially, this increase in growth and body size seems nothing but good, although the loss of taste of the overgrown vegetables, and the diseases which have increased as human stature has increased in the last decades in the most prosperous countries, should have warned that something was wrong.

In the stampede for quantity, a basic biological principle has been forgotten, namely, that any plant or animal has a specific size and weight, written down in its genetic constitution, the result of a long evolution. Only within this range of size is optimal efficiency or health possible. Insufficiency or excess are bound to levy a physiological price. In the course of evolution, insufficiency has occurred frequently enough for animals to become equipped with guidelines of reaction, in restlessness and hunger—plants, alas, cannot move. But excess has been so rare, that neither plants nor animals have any defences against it. Fed to excess, they get bigger and bigger, the physiological tax increasing proportionately. As the yield and the size of plants have been artificially stimulated, so the plant disease and the plant parasites have increased, calling for an ever increasing array of the most poisonous chemicals in an attempt to control the scourge. In animals and men, the excessive stimulation of growth has also been attended by an increasing recourse to drugs of one kind or another.

Just as over-fed rats get bigger and suffer increasingly from heart disease, diabetes, kidney disease, liver disease, so do humans. Athletes appear particularly prone to certain diseases, and their life-span is less than average, not because of the physical strain they subject themselves to—the body

47

thrives on that—but because of their thoroughly abnormal and excessive feeding.

It is undeniable that chronic malnutrition since the Dark Ages in Europe, led to a stunting of the population. The over-fed privileged classes were probably oversized, a factor no doubt in their often brutal domination of the masses. While it is difficult to define the specific range of the human species—racial difference are important—it is in all likelihood significantly less than the size attained by the so called 'best fed' nations, which has increased for a century as the quantity of animal foods increased in the diet.

Plant breeding has been size and calorie conscious. Foods new to the West, high in calories like the potato, and sugar, joined in the rush for quantity, much helped by a cheapening of flour by refining, with the result that, by the close of the nineteenth century, the masses in the industrial countries not only ate to their full, but had become gluttons, over-eating daily.

The evil of the new abundance in calorie foods lies in the excessive provision of calories without a sufficiency of the other essentials, the vitamins and minerals, many of them needed for the efficient use of the calories. So it is that foods like white flour and sugar, and indeed potato and other preponderantly starchy foods, can only be properly metabolized by tapping into the body's reserves of certain vitamins and minerals. When these reserves run low, zeal and efficiency fall, and ultimately, disease results.

With the new abundance, in a few decades, diseases which had formerly largely attacked the privileged, became the common affliction of the masses—diseases of the blood vessels, of the heart, strokes, kidney diseases, and the increasing list of diseases associated with over-weight. While this abundance gives to youth a greater appearance of health in increased stature, maturity and old age are increasingly associated with the functional, degenerating diseases, of which cancer and heart disease now claims the largest number of victims. But the young are also becoming affected by such disease.

48

Although hygiene overcame premature death due to infections, and so increased the life-span from the beginning of the nineteenth century, the virus diseases have increased steadily. The virus barely deserves the designation of being alive: it is no more than a minute cluster of protein molecules, very closely related to the DNA and RNA proteins manufactured by the genes in the cells of all plants and animals. There is increasing evidence that viruses can arise within the body, owing to faulty manufacture of RNA by the genes. Once manufactured, they continue replicating their kind by forcing the genes of other cells to manufacture the mistake that brought them into being, so that viruses assume an apparent independence. The demarcation between unnatural virus and natural gene is becoming all the more blurred, as the protein processes of the cell are unravelled. It may well turn out that viruses are the result of faulty protein metabolism, which could mean faulty protein feeding. It is certainly striking that as the amount of high protein animal foods has increased in the diet of the prosperous communities, so have the virus diseases. Some cancers are now suspected of being virus induced.

Although the eye is easily deceived by size, assuming that large size is the right size, many people are now sensing the deception. This illusion is a part of the quantity bias of quantity-geared, materialistic industrial civilization. Once sensitivity is restored, there is an inherent aversion to the oversized, just as the oversized flowers produced by horticulturists are felt by the more sensitive to be vulgar and monstrous. There is a 'feel' about the large fruits and vegetables which is wrong. Perhaps those closer to the soil have retained something of this sensitivity, for the more canny farmers do not use chemicals or insecticides on the crops they will consume themselves. More people are realizing that the risk of a maggot is preferable to an invisible puff of arsenic.

Until the full momentum of the industrial revolution was felt in the furthest lands, the varieties of human dietary were

49

infinite. Some were no doubt as deviant as the modern diet, but many others were more humanly compatible. In many parts of the world, especially in the more congenial and benevolent environments, human beings abandoned the ways acquired in the Ice Ages for patterns of life closer to the human norm, in soil-respecting farming communities and in peaceful relationship with their neighbours. This was largely the case in India before the population stampede and nutritional failures of modern times, in the Polynesian islands, among the native tribes of South America. Possibly these more gentle and humane peoples escaped the worst onslaught of the Ice Ages; the full anger against nature seems to be particular to the more Northern peoples, in Europe as in the Far East, and it is these peoples, particularly the Europeans, who are responsible for what has become an unwhole, and a denaturing planetary civilization.

It is this planetary influence which is so distressing, for the few remaining instances of a more humanizing situation are being rapidly assaulted. Soon, there will be no evidence left of a once happier and fairer condition. The deleterious influence of the West on the more benign peoples of the earth, in the guise of colonialism, of warfare, of alcoholism, of commercial exploitation, of disease, is well known. What is as yet not realized, is that the gluttony of the West, which may well have fed its restlessness and anger, and so prompted its planetary dominance, has been largely paid for by the misappropriation of planetary resources and the further impoverishment of the poorer peoples of the earth.

10. The Impoverishments of Prosperity

The Industrial Revolution was preceded, and has been accompanied, by a frantic commercial adventuring, which has brought the European with his trading practices all over the world. The essential feature of European trading is the exclusive priority it places on profits. Profitability has conditioned, and still conditions, practice, often at the detriment of the less easily definable human values. The introduction of rice refining in India is an example. Previously, the removal of the husk, the sifting away of the chaff, left much of the germ behind, the ritualized preoccupation of women, a labour of love and gratitude. Mildew, insects and rats no doubt took a considerable toll of the rice stores, but this was taken as one of the inevitables of existence; the rats also had a right to live! The European influence brought in quite another mentality, and a new class of European and Indian merchants, who set about correcting these wastes, by proper storage following the refining of the rice. In an age when the merits of hygiene were being widely promoted, white rice could be put over as a superior, cleaner product; with the losses due to spoilage overcome, the refined rice could be sold more cheaply while still leaving large profits to the merchants.

There was at first much resistance against these changes, which the Indian felt was a dismantling of a ritualized act of immense importance, but cheapness, and the withdrawal of whole rice by the merchants, forced the habit upon the Indian masses, aided perhaps by the fact that the European, because of his 'mixed diet', found the fibreless white rice more congenial to his taste. But the consequences were soon calamitous. Deficiencies of the B vitamins had been virtually unknown in India before. Now they became rampant, affecting whole communities, resulting in an apathy which in return affected the labour available to the colonial powers. An attempt was made, as soon as it was realized that the essential vitamins were contained in the endosperm and germ, to remedy this state of affairs by parboiling the rice before it was refined. Thereby some of the B vitamins penetrated the white grain. This not only added to the cost of the eventual product, but left behind an unpleasant soggy taste and smell. When the British Government attempted to make the eating of parboiled rice compulsory, there were riots.

The effect of rice refining in India, as elsewhere, has been utterly disastrous, leading to a chronic malnutrition that has debased the enterprise and the viability of the people. It is unfortunately true that a vegetarian is all the more damaged by eating refined cereals than a mixed eater, for the latter obtains considerable amounts of the B vitamins from the animal ingredient in his diet, whereas the vegetarian depends very largely on the B vitamins in cereals.

Sugar is another example of an impoverishment in the name of technical progress. By itself, sugar should not be considered a food. Although the natural fuel of all animal life, it is offered in nature with other essentials—particularly Vitamin C in the case of fruits—and is intended to be part of a whole dietary which supplies the essentials needed by the body for the proper metabolism of sugar, chiefly the B vitamins and certain minerals. Taken by itself, sugar is an anti-food. In combination with other refined foods, deprived of the B vitamins and minerals, it becomes a pernicious and evil ingredient in the diet, especially in one already inadequate and impoverished, the case in many parts of the world today.

It is depressing to contemplate how a delightful inducement, the primate love of sweetness, which is the natural demand for fruits, should have become so deceived, with deleterious consequences only now becoming better understood. Besides the well established responsibility for dental caries, sugar has recently been incriminated in a particular form of listlessness in children, often with fit-like attacks and destructive behaviour, seriously affecting the ability of such children to learn and to behave in a socially constructive manner. Sugar has been also invoked in heart attacks, in diseases of the skin and eye, in diabetes and other metabolic disturbances, as well as being the main contributor to the diseases of overweight.

Although other questionable crops, such as the vine, are grown on lands often inappropriate to the production of primary foods, beet sugar has become an established rotational crop on some of the best lands in Europe. Easy to grow and profitable, the acreage under beet has had to be limited, but it is a perversion of land use to grow sugar beet at all. Its place could be better taken by other rotational crops which could be used as a primary food. As for cane sugar, it is true that it is the most efficient means of fixing solar energy —were it not for the present clamour for sugar, converted into alcohol it could rival petrol at present prices—but human food is much more than calories. With the increasing world pressure on the primary foods, there is no doubt that the cane producing lands would do better to grow primary foods rather than sugar—less cars and gadgets, and less foreign exchange, but better health, and a happier people.

But it is the use of lands, capable of growing primary human foods like cereals, for meat production, that constitutes the greatest economic folly. It requires some twelve to fifteen times more land to produce a pound of meat than a pound of cereal, which means that some two to three thousand million more people could be fed if the world became vegetarian. It is not suggested that the world population should so increase. Rather, the aim is to emphasize how wasteful it has become to use land for the production

53

of animal food, a wastefulness which the planet can no longer tolerate.

Since the power of demand is still largely in the hands of the industrial communities, and their clamour for meat, far from being satiated, is for ever increasing, and since much of the animal feeding stuffs is produced in the poorer parts of the world, it means that the nutrition of the poorer two thirds of the planet is being increasingly sacrificed so that the gluttony of the more prosperous communities can be met. One can doubt that such a situation will be tolerated for much longer, for more than oil, the West has been meeting its protein surfeits at the expense of a planetary majority.

The situation is already threatening. The shortage of animal food is boosting prices, a main factor in the inflationary costs of feeding. Those countries formerly exporting animal foods are now consuming it themselves. And there is no unexploited land left on the planet. If the industrial communities do succeed in even maintaining their present levels of consumption of animal foods, it can only be at the cost of a deteriorating world situation, leading inexorably to worldwide starvation. And starving people are desperate people. With the means of making atomic weapons now well within the capacity of the poorer, increasingly more poorly fed peoples of the world, it is not impossible that the planetary holocaust will be the result of greed.

Wisdom would conclude that a worldwide adoption of a vegetarian dietary is the proper means of planetary justice and survival. Wisdom would also prepare for this inevitable change in good time, so that it came about in good order, without the widespread disaster which such momentous change will exact if it comes about in violence and chaos. Unfortunately, it is not only the greed of the presently prosperous countries that is involved. Many of the poorer peoples have come to imitate the dietary habits of the West, as they have attempted to catch up with its industrial advantages. Former peasantries, only eating animal foods on rare festive occasions, now insist on a daily intake, as the mark of emancipation. And many of the poorer peoples are, by culture and tradition, the opposite of vegetarian.

The prospects are undoubtedly grim. Success is only likely to be achieved if the overall bad habits of civilization, as well as the mounting pressure of population, can become corrected. In all probability, all these problems are interconnected. Wrong eating must in some way at present unrealized, play its part in the population stampedes of recent times, just as this stampede has its reverse influence on world food resources. The challenge of a world food reform calls for a better understanding of the forces at work behind the extraordinary rise in the human population of this planet.

11. The Unloving Crowd

Although the earth could support a considerably larger number of people than exist at present on a vegetarian dietary, congestion is fast becoming a dehumanizing influence. Human society differs from the often vast aggregations of individuals one finds among other animals, wherein the individual is subordinate to the group structure, in that society is the radiation of the humanizing predispositions engendered within each individual. It is only when such conditions are fulfilled in the individual that society is itself a humanizing force. Constraint, limitation of individual freedom, subordination of the individual to the needs of vast societies are thus inherently antihuman.

Human love is so powerful a force, that it can no doubt be exercised in large social groupings, possibly extending to a planetary scale. But this requires first of all the reality of love and its achievement between individuals, as well as a social structure which preserves individual liberty, in the sense of allowing and encouraging every individual to develop along humanizing lines. Unfortunately, the larger the social groupings in human history, the greater the interferences in such liberty. The rise of the first civilizations were attended by such dehumanizing devices as slavery, and although slavery has been condemned for over a hundred years, human beings have become increasingly subordinate to the vast social groups, with the crises of coercion expressed in the totalitarian regimes.

Under such conditions, humanization is thwarted. If

human beings are not thugs and bullies, they become passive and uncaring, which is a form of dehumanization. But the effects of overcrowding, inevitable with the rise of the gigantic modern metropolis, are more insidious. Even in rats, spared the precarious balance of the human mind, over-crowding results in antihuman parallels—in killing and maiming without reason, in a neglect of the young, in queer sexual practices, and in inexplicable bursts of communal madness. In its over-plentifulness, human life is becoming dangerously cheap. The calculations of over-kill, in the event of a nuclear war, are symptomatic of such cheapening.

Quite apart from the increasing pressure on the resources offered by nature, the impact of overcrowding on the environment has the antihuman consequence of leading to a disorderly, ugly environment. This is evident enough even where order prevails—in architecture, where the pressure of economics and maximal utilization of space has filled the cities with concrete and glass boxes devoid of human meaning. Where the population pressure results in a breakdown of order, the results are appalling, in the clutter and dirt of modern cities, in the noise and enervating bustle, in the congestions of crowd and traffic, in the pollution of the air, in the loss of sunlight, not to mention those hideous consequences of urban disorder, the slums and semi-slums that fester around all cities, and increasingly within them.

As the crowded cities have spread, forever consuming more of the countryside, so nature has become increasingly devastated, and rendered meaningless. It is one of the most depressing observations to find the degree to which city inhabitants, including the young, come to lose all contact with nature, to the point where they feel lost and awkward, if not actually listless and violent, when brought into contact with what is precariously left of nature. The fact is that unless nature is free and uncorrupted, it does lose much of its meaning to the human being. For one thing, the sense of an invigorating purity one can experience in unspoilt and beautiful scenes, is ruled out—by as little as a carelessly discarded wrapper! Since the appreciation of purity, as much as beauty and harmony, are essential humanizing attributes, this loss of environmental purity results in an impure human being, necessarily more callous, more able to accept the hideousness of the environment in which he finds himself.

Anthropologists are agreed about few things, but most of them concur that large-scale conflict—what has come to be known as war—is a relatively recent occurrence. It has increased in severity and extent, and in its dehumanization, as population pressure has increased. What then is the reason for this extraordinary soaring in the human population, itself a recent phenomenon? If the human species has existed for hundreds of thousands of years, and a human-like primate for millions, this crisis of over-population is all the more extraordinary.

The hominids of the Palaeolithic roamed over most of the world. If it was only a matter of food, then surely they would have stumbled upon conditions in some part of the world where the kind of rapid increase we are witnessing would have occurred. All the evidence indicates that the hominids, like the higher primates, have never known a population explosion. They have been as a group, restricted breeders. Gorillas and chimpanzees maintain stable populations; overcrowding only comes from human encroachment into their habitats. It cannot be disease, in the form of the sweeping and devastating epidemics known in the crowded and unsanitary conditions of the urban past, that kept their numbers down, for the surviving bands of gorillas, already seriously menaced by human intrusion, are superbly healthy.

One way in which population stability is maintained in such primates, is by varying the length of nurture. Nursing mothers are not sexually harassed by the males, so that if nurture is prolonged, the occasions for breeding are reduced. The males are not inconvenienced, for although ever-ready to mount a receptive female, they only become sexually aroused on signals of one kind or another from the females, and can spend a life of bachelor uninvolvement if no such signals come.

More usually, nursing persists long enough after birth to cut down the breeding cycles for a particular female so that not more than a few offspring result. With the hazards of babyhood in the wild, this maintains a stable population. If the population increases, mothers nurture their young for longer, to such an extent that the number of offspring can be considerably reduced. In all primates, including the human, there is in fact a clash between the hormones involved in suckling and nursing, and those of breeding, so that the female has no interest in sex during nurture, a device of obvious biological advantage, for if female mammals were more interested in sex than in breeding, the line would have become extinct early, an interest which little girls with their little dolls still demonstrate, no matter how they behave later.

Is the human an exception to this primate breeding control. Could it not be that the stampede of over population is the outcome of a deranged breeding pattern, as abnormal as the patterns of eating and sex already mentioned? It is commonly assumed, with the support of scientific authority, that the human female has lost the cyclical nature of the oestral cycle, and thereby the female decision regarding the time of coitus. The human female is described as 'open'. This is a cultural falsification, a device to provide the human male with the ready access to sexual relief he has come to require, for there is definite evidence that women have a peak desire for coitus during the oestral cycle, which implies that it is in such peaks that the woman would best accept the man. In thus complying with the other primates, it would follow that the woman would also follow the primate device of extending nurture as a means of population control.

The way in which the natural woman would do this is probably through the pituitary gland. As population pressure increases, so the social environment becomes less assured, anxiety increases, and child care intensified. It requires no conscious observation, no reasoning. Intuitively, the woman senses the threat of population pressure to the species. There is some indication that primitive groups, such as those in the Amazon basin, had achieved stability by such means, before the interruptions of civilized men. But it is to be noted that this control depends on a sufficient degree of human sensitivity, both on the part of the woman, in order to sense intuitively the social situation, and on the part of the man to respect her increased preoccupation with child nurture. A loss of sensitivity, and the device breaks down.

The situation is complicated by the fact that the woman, unlike the other primate females, is largely conditioned by her cortex. If she exists in a society wherein the woman is considered 'open', so she acts, and believes herself to be open to male whim and fancy. This is true also regarding the orgasm, which is an essentially male preoccupation forced upon the general sexual pattern, to the point where orgasmically harassed women become bad mothers, failing in what is after all the pre-eminent female biological duty. The fact of the situation is that while nature has placed the essential responsibility of breeding on the female, it is the male in the human situation who has come to decide the sexual pattern, and this pattern is essentially geared to male sexual pleasure, freed from the entanglements of love, and even of breeding care, which is as good a definition of lust as one can find.

Rejecting the existential evidence, one can suppose that humanization occurred in humanly congenial conditions, and that sexual restraint on the part of the male was a natural human ability, not the psychological liability it has been claimed to be, in which case the size of the human population in terms of the environment would be controlled as it is in other primates—by a greater preoccupation with breeding and less with sex. Under existential conditions, the reverse seems to apply; the more anxious and harassing the times, the more people breed. Evidently, something has happened which has inflamed sexual desire, to the point where it overrides the biological perimeters of the species, and this something may well be traceable to the amines already mentioned as originating in a faulty and inhuman diet, combined with a general humanizing impoverishment characteristic of civilization. Premature sexual interests in children can often be simply traced to wrong feeding, especially in animal foods.

Since the Ice Ages, the abnormal amines have been affecting the mind, but on the whole, human beings have not become beset by a demented sexual urge. A hard life, and a hard faith, no doubt helped. In fact, in early times, human breeding may have been so restrained, that religion intervened to boost breeding in order to meet a changed society, one increasingly determined by a more congested existence. The stampede only got under way with the rise of civilization, and its adverse effect of sexual love, combined with an increase in the pathological stimulation of the lower aspects of the mind. The incidence of child neglect and of promiscuity, indicate the severity of the dementia. With some 18 per cent of births the result of transient unions in the big cities of civilization, and a much higher proportion of unloved children, the condition is an advanced one, threatening human survival.

Food has been in league with this situation, for unless the food supplies were increased to meet the ever-increasing harvest of babies, population control would have been long ago affected by starvation and pestilence. So it is that intensive agriculture, the abuse of artificial fertilizers, the mechanization of meat, milk and egg production, the adulteration, refining and preservation of food, the intensifying exploitation of the oceans, and the complex chemical and poisonous paraphernalia of civilized food technology are as guilty as lust, the reverse side of the same counterfeit coin.

12. The Deceits of Lucullus

When one considers that all other animals consume food as nature presents it to them, and that virtually no food is now eaten in a natural condition, one is entitled to ask how such an extraordinary recourse to artificiality could have arisen. It is not always hunger that drives people to eat the extraordinary foods like maggots, birds' nests, barnacles and tripe, but some curious perversion of taste, and the endless, often unnecessary adulterations and interferences with foods point to a related assault against the simple and natural, symptoms of man's revulsion against the natural world.

The artificialities of food, the endless search for the titillation of a jaded palate, are also the results of frustration and boredom. Lucullus was a Roman general who never lost a battle, but was eventually betrayed by the politicians at home. In disgust, he retired to gourmandize, inventing sumptuous dishes and gastronomic orgies never before imagined, with an army of cooks instead of centurions. Faced with the frustrations of living some people take to the way of Lucullus. The business magnate gorges himself to death, not because he is successful, but because he is humanly frustrated, secretly cheated of meaning and value to life, in the ruthless acquisitiveness of a materialistic jungle. As a result, since the Romans, and in fact long before them, there has been a succession of able food inventors and artificers.

Such enticements to gluttony become self-perpetuating. The glutton's preoccupation with food has much the same features as that of the compulsive addict, with ever more varied and outrageous titillations needed, until the ludicrous is reached as in the food fantasies of Lucullus. Fire was probably first used for cooking in order to overcome the nauseating smell and taste of raw meat and it was used by the early food collectors to soften the hard fibres of vegetable foods that could not be eaten raw. For a long, long time, cooking was thus primarily utilitarian. It was only with the use of more sophisticated culture that the cook became an acrobat.

The softening of vegetable fibres enables vegetables to be better digested in a mixed diet. Over-coarse vegetable foods interfere with protein absorption and result in putrefaction, nausea and general gastric disquiet which can end in an actual dislike of all vegetables, commonly observed in big flesh eaters. This explains why many people insist that vegetables which can perfectly well be eaten raw, be thoroughly cooked. But a price is paid for this emasculation of vegetable food. Not only the common constipation, but more serious diseases like diverticulitis result from a prolonged insufficiency of vegetable fibres in the diet.

The softening of the food also enables the normal mechanism of satiety to be cheated. A slice or two of wholemeal bread will induce a feeling of satisfaction, while a whole loaf of white bread still leaves a sense of dissatisfaction. The extraordinary ability of the stomach to expand is no doubt a natural provision enabling the primate to gorge when food is abundant; but this is rarely the case in nature, so that the stomach is not continuously distended to its fullest, as it is among the civilized. Big eaters have the highest incidence of stomach cancer.

There are also stimulants in abnormal foods, such as meat, which cause the stomach to over-secrete. Many hours after a meal of meat, peristaltic contractions persist, even when the stomach contents have emptied into the duodenum. It is these contractions which account for the common 'hunger pangs', a pathological demand for more food due to wrong feeding, often exacerbated by spices added to foods. Unlike appetite, this is not pleasant; relief only comes, transiently, as more food is taken in, a vicious circle at times leading to a visibly pathological gorging.

The real reason why many people prefer cooked to raw food is that it is much easier to overeat the cooked. Romans insisted on over-cooked foods, for they were easier to re-gurgitate. Hot food is also easier to abuse of than cold. When the overworked stomach cries for mercy, and seizes up when given cold food, it will be induced to open out with hot food, one more device for fooling nature. The insistence on 'piping hot' dishes is a sure sign that the natural gastric functions have been thoroughly sabotaged, the stomach, an over-irritated, beaten, humiliated organ, capable of accepting any abuse. The association of ulceration and cancer with hot, particularly fried food, seems clear.

Boiling not only softens vegetable fibres and overcomes the reek of raw animal food, but subtly alters proteins, dissolves out minerals, and makes the starches and sugars more quickly absorbable, by no means an advantage, for the continuous flooding of the blood with too easily absorbed sugars is probably the cause of an ultimate breakdown of sugar metabolism, resulting in diabetes, in abnormal fat deposition in tissues, in blood vessel degeneration, especially when combined with saturated animal fats. But frying is undoubtedly much worse, for heat forms extremely irritating substances, many of which are carcinogenetic. The oil used again and again in restaurant kitchens, in many fish-and-chip shops, is as potent a cancer producing brew as one can find in any laboratory.

The art of cooking means replacing the natural flavours lost by the action of heat, of solution, of dissipation and storage, and today, of intensive agriculture and the industrial-ization of food production. A battery of flavours, spices, con-diments is always ready to hand in every kitchen. But it is salt which is the pivot of gastronomy, so much so, that everyone accepts that salt is a natural and necessary addition to food. Since the basal needs of salt are no more than two or three grams, and most people add twenty to thirty times this amount to their daily foods, one is evidently dealing with a dietary perversion. Salt craving in man and in animals is probably the craving for minerals, due to a deficiency in the food, or disease, when the body can waste phenomenal amounts of minerals. In nature, animals drawn to the rare saltlicks are invariably diseased. Normal animals will not touch salt, although salt hunger is common in animals associated with man, no doubt due to mineral-defective food. In the human diet, mineral deficiency is most probably due to losses in cooking. Raw foods often have a discernible mineral tang, which is rapidly lost in cooking. There is a further reason in the fact that if salt is added to the food, the body is so disturbed as to become very wasteful of it, often overspilling large amounts of salt in the urine and sweat. Animal foods are rich in salt, so that on a mixed diet, even without added salt, there is a mineral disturbance, leading to salt craving. It is at last becoming realized that the common, virtually universal abuse of salt is incriminated in a long list of diseases, more particularly involving the heart, the kidneys, changes in the lens of the eye, blood pressure and oedema.

Cooking has not only facilitated the eating of animal foods, but has enabled the eating of many food articles which could not be eaten in a raw condition, a fact which should make any such food suspect in the first place, however palatable it may become after cooking and preparation. Take the case of the potato. Available in Europe from the sixteenth century, it played a leading part in the population increases. Not only is it unpleasant in the raw, but it contains a poisonous alkaloid, which is enormously increased during the formation of the 'eyes' in storage. This alkaloid, solanin, reduces the oxygenerating capacity of the blood, blocks enzyme systems, and poisons the nerves. Recently it was discovered with considerable alarm, that foetuses could be permanently damaged if pregnant mothers ate spoiled or germinating

65

potatoes. Possibly all members of the solanum group should be considered suspect, for all have alkaloids, some immediately fatal, such as deadly nightshade. That the Aztecs ate large quantities of solanum vegetables is hardly a recommendation.

In the case of spinach or rhubarb, cooking shows how dangerous foods can be made so palatable as to be eaten to excess. Man is not ideally adapted to most mature green leaves, but rather to tender shoots, and in moderation, for shoots are not over-abundant in nature. Some shoots, however, and many mature leaves, have large amounts of oxalic acid, which the liver cannot efficiently metabolise. When eaten, the acid base balance of the body is threatened, calcium mobilized and wasted. In the raw state, such foods are unpleasantly acid, and no more than a bite would be taken. Cooked, dressed with butter and béchamel, spinach becomes delectable and rhubarb delicious, good examples of the dangers of gastronomy. Children, however, are often wiser, for in spite of such subterfuge, they appear to have an innate aversion to such foods.

Many people would be prepared to defend the art of cooking for the pleasure that it brings to a usually boring and frustrated existence. Unfortunately, these pleasures are transitory. After many a good meal, the bodily disquiet is all too apparent, in the flushed face and the beating heart. Only a few lucky people get away with it for any time. Usually, the price is paid depressingly early, when one should still be in the prime of life, at fifty, sixty, young still for a creature evidently designed for a very long existence. The trouble is that most people cannot conceive that simple, natural foods can afford pleasure. Only an overall reform of life attitudes, a revival of the meaning of purity, of beauty, can enable the sensing of the arcadean joys to be had in natural eating.

Natural eating does not mean crude, unattractive, unimaginative eating. On the contrary, the natural appeals of natural food can be enormously extended, if not by cooking, by presentation and preparation. The raw components need not be limited and dull, and with a minimum amount of cooking, a thoroughly satisfactory and humanly enhancing diet presents itself. The art of it remains, and has the beauty and purity which all art should bestow upon the human. By comparison, the art devices of gastronomy are no different from the false beauty of lipstick and pancake makeup.

13. The Costs of Confusion

Living in an age when the human being is looked upon as an accidental production of a Universe without meaning, subject to a nature prone to catastrophe, man is seen as no more than a cunning, randy naked ape. It would seem reasonable that people should grab for the immediate pleasures and satisfactions that existence can provide, without asking too many questions, particularly those involving right or wrong, good or bad. Philosophers themselves, who in the past have preoccupied themselves with the ideal, have come to the conclusion that only existence counts, that ideals are one more manifestation of illusion.

For those who believe that man is naturally an idealizing creature, however opportunistic and existentialistic he may appear, the modern situation can only be interpreted as the crisis of blindness and atrophy brought about by long ages of confusion, originally initiated by nature's own hostilities in the trials of the Ice Ages, but perpetuated ever since by an inability to feel and think clearly again. After many thousands of years of endeavouring to find the lost wisdom of which every one feels his due, the modern age has come to accept the impossibility of wisdom. It is a tragic situation, all the more tragic in that science has come to confirm the apparent futility of man.

Although most people do not like the effort involved in feeling and thinking deeply about such problems, and prefer to take life as it comes, clearly the way out of the present confusions, with their roots in the most distant past, can only be found by some very deep and passionate thinking indeed. In facing the problem examined in this book—the question of right eating—a practical resolution it not enough. To have any effect, it must be backed by belief that man has meaning, that essence is what primarily matters, for existence can only have meaning when it complies with essence, with the rules set by nature for human existence, the opposite of the usual opportunism.

The problem is a circuitous one; living existentially, one comes to believe that only existence matters. In the case of food and feeding, it is simply not felt possible that there can be any ideal pattern; like all things, food is an occasion for the natural opportunist scramble. It is generally believed that the gory, gluttonous, promiscuous Primal Horde is only held down by social censure, by the primitive law of an eye for an eye, and today, law and censure in themselves are being dismantled in a rising, officially backed opportunism. We have all become petty criminals, and no longer much troubled by the fact.

This turn of events is not only disastrous in its inhuman consequences, but is irrational, for the most elementary lesson that biology should have to teach is that nature not only favours the fit and eliminates the unfit, but rewards only the fit, mercilessly punishing the unfit. This does not depend on any ulterior meaning or morality in the working of nature. It is a purely practical, indispensable provision in the functioning of things. If reward and punishment are not a built-in provision, as fundamental as the particular ways in which atoms combine with one another to form the myriad substances of nature and of living things, the whirling clouds of hydrogen gas, which appeared at the beginning of the universe some fifteen billion years ago, would still be whirling around, having accomplished nothing.

Modern existentialism has been the work of thinkers with no scientific training. Scientists, biologists in particular, could easily dismantle their systems; their guilt should be that so few of them have had the courage to speak out against the falsities of so many of the widely advertised and accepted conclusions of the age. Accepting that nature works on the principles of rewards and punishments, it should be evident that the modern opportunist, existentialistic attitudes cannot possibly bring genuine gratification. If there are apparent pleasures in the purely random ways in which people live, then they can but amount to illusions, certain to carry a backwash of retribution. The impartial examination of any aspect of modern living shows this to be true, whether it be politics or sex, medicine or feeding. The apparent rewards of power invariably bring with them the attendants of insensitivity, and the joys of so called freedom in sex disappointments and painfulness. The trouble is that so hollow has life become, that people will not face the emptiness of the only rewards to living which they believe exist, the pleasures of the palate, of the bed, of money, of material gadgetry and power, of the bogus communalism of urban living, of the mechanically expressed restlessness of the disturbed modern soul.

So it is that most people would probably contend that the satisfactions of the ordinary life, admitting that they involve many departures from normality, are worth the while, the price worth paying, if indeed there is a price at all. Almost everyone believes that it is not all that important what one eats, as long as one has variety and amount enough. There has to be something very wrong with a meal for one to be punished with a stomach ache. Uncomplainingly, the body accepts the legions of daily transgressions of a lesser kind without protest. When catastrophe eventually occurs— and many appear to escape altogether—in a burst blood vessel, in a seizing arthritic joint, the long abuse of natural law seems quite inapparent. Bad luck, accident, nature's inherent imperfections seem the more likely causes.

But if the majority are the victims of such confusion, it seems hardly believable that science, and medicine in particular, do not more frequently protest against the common waywardness. Over the past two or three decades, the evidence has been mounting, enough to leave no doubt that man's misfortunes are largely self-inflicted, by carelessness, by greed, by stupidity, and that the price paid in suffering is astronomical. Science clearly serves the particular culture in which it exists; it is no independent impartial overseer.

The common assumption that disease is 'natural' and naturally inevitable, the consequences of a wayward and imperfect nature, to be remedied only by human interference, is at the heart of much of the confusion. One must admit that nature is not perfect, but nature does quite often achieve perfection, even if to appreciate the refinements of this perfection, one has to go beyond the realm of appearances, as science has discovered. As insisted upon in the course of this book, humanization must have occurred initially under ideal conditions, even if things went wrong subsequently. Health and happiness should therefore be natural possibilities, provided the original humanizing conditions can be restored.

For transgressions which have recurrently occurred in the history of life, the cataclysms of climate and food change, of earth movements, of floodings and dessications, living things have an inexhaustible reservoir of experience to call upon. Given time, readaptation to change follows, and the animal survives. But if the transgression is unnatural, as in the case of laboratory or industrial products, there is not only a complete absence of past experience to be drawn upon, but no symptom of distress following the ingestion of such substances, for symptoms to some offending agent take millions of years to evolve. So it is that the causes of the most terrible, life-destroying diseases remain ignored, and syptomless, calling for no readjustments, until the body is literally overwhelmed, as is the case in many cancers.

Today, every contact with the environment is contaminated with such unnatural substances. A recent attempt to draw up a list of such substances ran into tens of thousands. Every year, hundreds are being added. The official attitude to such a dangerous situation—that a substance cannot be condemned until it is proved harmful—shows a complete disdain of biological principles. Those relying on this test are mostly guilty men, often aware of the harm ultimately likely, but more concerned with expediency than with human wholeness.

It is often contended that the situation cannot be as bad as the pessimists claim, for has not the human life span been extensively increased, and are not many, once crippling diseases conquered? Medical and scientific journalists, often not scientists themselves, are in the habit of hinting that such achievements are thanks to science's conquest over nature's natural infirmities, implying that the 'natural' life-span has been extended, that a naturally sick nature has been corrected. This is biological nonsense. Every species of animal has a genetically set life-span, a setting closely related to its rate of growth. If this correlation is applied to man, the most slowly developing of all creatures, then the human life-span should be well over a hundred years. All that science has in fact achieved is the removal of unsanitary conditions and the control of diseases inherent in such conditions. The unhealthiness of Ice Age Palaeolithic humans can be seen in the pathological torturings of their bones, but the worst ravages of unhealthiness probably only came with the urbanization of living, in the earliest civilizations. There are hints that when the Ice Ages ended, and before the rise of the first civilizations, human beings lived long, whole lives, a length which has not been fully recovered. There are still isolated peasantries in which many individuals live well over the century. Quite recently, as the functional collapse intensifies in soaringly degenerative diseases, the cancers and heart diseases in particular, there has been a dip in the life-span. Far from confidence in the apparent successes of science and medicine, there should be alarm, for while the diseases that have been corrected, due to pathogenic organisms, only affect individuals, the degenerative diseases entail a definite genetic impoverishment.

Here again, one is faced with a barrage of propaganda,

optimistic and pontifical, that some success has been achieved, that cancers can be cured. But for one case surviving a number of years after operation and treatment, dozens die, for all the vast agitations of worldwide research. Some cancers undoubtedly begin quite locally, as in the case of radiation damage, and if removed in time, survival is assured. But in most cases, the localized appearance of a cancer is only a stage in what is a general underlying pathology, involving the entire body, so evident in the leukaemias. Medicine has yet to admit that most diseases of such a nature are not localized, but entail a failure of the entire organism, an admission which would entail a revolution in medical philosophy, away from its present mechanical concepts, to more holistic ones. There are at the moment indications that something in this direction is happening, in the admission that exercise and diet are the best ways of preventing heart attacks, that years of over-eating are likely to end in diabetes, and that possibly the best if not the only way of combating many kinds of cancer is through the body's own abilities to react. But evidently, before there can be a real change of heart, there has to be a fundamental change in ideology, in the world-view of science, in its attitudes to man and nature, and judging the slowness of progress in this direction, one can be excused for doubting that there is sufficient survival time.

14. Food Fit for Humans

Basing oneself on the humanizing aesthetic criteria, and making use of the scientific evidence that complies with them, one can define the ideal human diet as one beautiful and refreshing, consisting of fruits in abundance, of seeds and nuts, of cereals and tender shoots and leaves, of flowers, eaten in the raw. Unfortunately, given the present-day interferences in natural foods, it is unlikely that such an ideal dietary is possible, for almost all foods available today, are produced from unnatural, variously disturbed soils. Sadly therefore, no longer is a purely simple wisdom adequate. This is where a science, serving the human condition rather than undermining it, can help.

Treating the soil as nothing but a physical medium is the result of a materialistic, mechanical attitude to life and nature generally. While at first this seemed justified by the enormously increased yields which resulted from chemical fertilizers, it has become ever more apparent that the soil is a living medium, seriously undermined by such crude stimuli, and that foods grown on such disturbed soils lack substances indispensable to animals.

Since the work of McCarrison in India over half a century ago, it has been known that organically defective soils produce crops with a lowered vitamin B content. One of these vitamins in particular, Vitamin B_{12}, is more or less completely absent in such crops. Vitamin B_{12} is an exceptional and extraordinary substance, still something of a mystery although its chemical nature is fully known. It is a complex amine, nitrocobolamine, containing an atom of cobalt in its molecule, the only use known of this metal in biological processes. It is only needed in unimaginably minute amounts, a few millionths of a gram being sufficient. If this minute amount is not supplied, however, the most serious, possibly irreparable damage is done to the nervous system, besides serious ill effects on the blood-forming tissues.

One can go a considerable time without any of this vitamin in the food, weeks or months, for the liver stores considerable amounts of it. As vegetable foods only contain fractional amounts of it, and many none at all, even when grown on natural soils—fruits do not have a trace of it—the body can evidently absorb amounts so small that they can easily pass chemical detection. Since so little is needed by the tissues, even in such small amounts, the liver can presumably build up a reserve—under ideal conditions. Primates like the gorilla, who are strictly vegetarian, and the other vegetarian animals, must accumulate their needs of vitamin B_{12} in this way, and even on deficient soils, cattle for instance, appear to derive sufficient vitamin B_{12}. It is probable that the micro-organisms which abound in the digestive tracts of these animals produce some of their needs of this vitamin.

In the human being, traces of vitamin B_{12} are probably also supplied by micro-organisms in the gut, but these micro-organisms require the kind of fermentative conditions typical of a vegetarian dietary. Experiments on Vegans have shown that while some evidently derive enough of the vitamin, others do not do so, and the explanation of this difference is not yet understood. It is evidently not only a matter of raw food; probably the quality of the food comes into it. Owing to this uncertainty, and given the worldwide disturbance of the soil, it would be well for strict vegetarians to take a few micrograms of vitamin B_{12} periodically, for instance, for one week per month.

With this one exception, the ideal human requirements from food can undoubtedly be met by a preponderantly raw vegetarian diet. If fruits are eaten several times a day—the one item which can be eaten between meals—the high levels

75

of vitamin C can be satisfied. Although in normal conditions of health, much of this vitamin C is excreted in the urine, it should not be looked upon as a waste, for the human tissues seem to function best when continuously bathed with this vitamin. If always sufficiently present, passing infections are likely to be resisted, although when infection does occur, truly enormous amounts of this vitamin become necessary, which can only be met by large amounts of fruit juice, or the taking of vitamin C as a supplement. This should not be looked upon as a substitute for fruits, for there are many things in fruits, ponderable and imponderable, apart from their beauty and flavour, which are necessary, but it would be shortsighted to refuse to make use of this synthetic vitamin, in order to raise the vitamin C level when this becomes necessary.

In the cooler regions, fruits are seasonally scarce and expensive. Provided sufficient raw vegetable food is eaten, there should be no harm in taking smaller amounts of vitamin C daily in pill form. The complete non-toxicity of this vitamin has been amply proven; indeed, apart from water, it is about the only substance whose range is so wide as to be non-toxic even in amounts several hundred times the normal requirement. Furthermore, it is easily metabolized and excreted when in excess without taxing in any way the alkaline reserves of the tissues. The only condition under which large doses of vitamin C are questionable is when large amounts of dairy products are eaten. The vitamin C, which is an acid, may form kidney stones by combining with the calcium in these products. But then as we shall claim, dairy products are not a part of normal human food.

In relation to their size, children need more food than adults. There is no need for so called 'protective' foods, high in protein, provided children can eat whole foods when ever hungry, and the calamitous sweets are kept away. Left to themselves, children will eat often, ignoring the regularity of meals favoured by adults, which is well and good. The meal regularity is in fact one more device for eating more, even when not hungry, for, like the dogs of Pavlov, meal times can become the means of a cortical conditioning which stimulates even a jaded and overtired stomach.

It is thoroughly misguided to give children such supplements as vitamin A and D, particularly in such disgusting and loathed forms as the fish liver oils. The body is designed to make its own needs of these vitamins, in the case of the vitamin A from the carotenoid pigments abundant in the colourful tissues of plants, and in the case of vitamin D, from light irradiation of the skin. Since both these vitamins are stored in the liver, occasional supplies will suffice. Except in the more extreme latitudes, where humans should not be living anyway, there is sufficient light to make vitamin D, provided sufficient skin surface is exposed. A clear indication that these vitamins should not be eaten as such, is the recent discovery that children who have been adminstered fish oils over a prolonged period have a lower I.Q. than other children.

Life is preponderantly water, and almost all land animals need a regular supply of it. On an ideal human diet, so much water is contained in the fruits and vegetables, that very little water is needed. The addition of salt and other unnatural items completely upsets the water balance; as every one knows, thirst can become obsessive after a heavy meal. The need for water increases in hot weather. Unlike appetite, thirst is a reliable guide of body needs; it is unwise to drink except when thirsty.

The universe is a whole, and all things aspire to wholeness. Food reflects the wholeness which is life; all the constituents are interdependent. One often finds that if a particular vitamin deficiency is treated, others previously not apparent become manifest. This means that when the ideal diet for any particular species of animal prevails, there is no need to fuss about proteins, calories, vitamins and minerals.

Some items of food, commonly consumed but doubtfully a part of the normal human dietary, will now be examined, with a view to ascertaining the physiological cost they entail. For some, the price is evidently too high; others have a certain value as emergency foods.

Milk. Generally considered a 'protective' food, except by the Chinese who look upon it as an obnoxious excrement. The milk of the different mammals varies considerably. The short-lived species have made no attempt to remove substances which could, over a number of years, jeopardise the longevity of the animal. So it is that cow's milk is high in those substances, the cholesterols and saturated fats, which slowly clutter up the blood vessels—cows and bulls do not live long enough for it to matter. In elephants, and in the higher primates, however, the composition of the milk is quite different. Not only is protein lower, but the saturated fats are replaced by less saturated and unsaturated, and the cholesterol is low. Furthermore, the first milk fed to infant elephants and primates, the colostrum, is particularly rich in unsaturated fats. It is now realized that the quality of the blood vessels is determined by the early feeding of the young; to give cow's milk to a baby elephant or a primate is to predispose its blood vessels and heart to lifelong damage by saturated fats. The autopsies of quite young people today show often extensive circulatory damage, most likely due to the common habit of drinking cow's milk from infancy.

Skim milk is less harmful, but one can doubt that the proteins of cow's milk are minutely identical to those of the human, the one needed for rapid growth, the other for slow development. Cream is a particularly dangerous food.

Margarine, made from soft vegetable fats by saturating them with hydrogen, is no better than butter, although they have little or no cholesterol, for their fat molecules are very much larger than those of human milk fat, and result in the deposition of fats as hard as those of animal food in the tissues. The soft margarines, made from partly hydrogenated vegetable fats, to which is added oils rich in unsaturated fats, are suspect, in view of the chemicals used in their manufacture, and of the reports of serious disease following their experimental use in animals. Vegetable 'butters' made from emulsified nuts should be excellent, provided no emulsifying or other chemical agents are used in their manufacture. If one likes some fat on one's bread, the ancient device of Mediterranean peasants of dripping a little olive oil on the bread, rubbed with a little garlic, is a good one.

Kephir, Yogourt, etc. Widely and anciently praised as a 'health' food, the fatty constituents remain much the same, although the growth of bacteria and yeasts, producing an acid medium, is favourable to anti-putrefactive conditions which should be helpful. But one should preferably not eat foods that putrefy. These preparations made with skimmed or defatted milk are preferable.

Cheese. Hippocrates had noticed that cheese adversely affects a significant number of people, an indication that it is not a natural food. It has recently been incriminated in migraine. The hard, fullfat cheeses are more suspect than the lighter kinds made with whey. At the most cheese should only be used occasionally, and in small amounts not so much as a food item but as a condiment.

Eggs are designed to meet the extremely rapid growth of reptiles and birds, and as such, are the opposite of human needs. Their extremely high content of cholesterol makes them a dangerous food, perhaps the most dangerous. Furthermore, they are the vehicle of many viruses, known and unknown.

Coffee, tea, chocolate. The popularity of these items comes not only from their stimulating properties, but from their very high content of purines and other extractives. On a 'mixed' diet, the body over-reacts against such extractives in the foods, thus engendering a drug-like demand for more, to mop up the body's over-production of defensive substances, resulting in a vicious circle of ever-increasing demand. If one must have hot drinks, many herbal teas are harmless. Weak tea seems less harmful than coffee.

Vegetable oils. Although the unsaturated fatty acid content of different vegetable oils varies, thus affecting their value for eliminating saturated fats from the body, no vegetable oil contains the saturated fats abundant in all animal oils. Therefore, on a vegetarian diet, it is a matter of taste what oil one prefers. Olive oil, for instance, has a low content of unsaturated fats, but is tasty and good. The only safe fats, however, are those that have been cold pressed, out of contact with metal contamination; it is virtually impossible to obtain such oils today. Commercial processes entail the use of dangerous solvents, and high temperature extraction responsible for undesirable changes in the oil itself, quite apart from anti-oxidant chemicals used to prevent rancidity.

One vegetable oil, rape seed oil, is toxic, and is being phased out of use. However, it is still the cheapest oil on the market. It is usually sold without a reference to its source, as just 'salad' or 'frying' oil, and is widely used in food processing and in restaurants.

Potatoes, cassavas and starchy roots. The toxicity of the alkaloids of potato have already been mentioned. Cassava contains deadly prussic acid and will rapidly kill when eaten raw. The real menace of such items is that they tend to reduce the consumption of cereals, which should be the main source of calories in combination with fruits.

Bread, biscuits

Fresh cereal grains can be nibbled like nuts, but once dried, something has to be done to them so that they can be eaten. The best way is to soak them and allow them to germinate. Germinating grains are about the richest sources of a battery of indispensable vitamins. Some should always be set to germinate in succession in some corner of the home, or office.

Soaked grains can be mashed, pounded and moulded into thin wafers, which can then be dried in a low oven, or yeast can be added, and the dough baked as bread. The damp conditions prevailing, and the moderate temperatures

80

necessary, are not critical. Lightly cooked groat or porridge, goes back to the Palaeolithic. Unfortunately, industrial production of bread and biscuits, even many classed as 'brown' or 'wholemeal', is highly suspect, so that the best answer is to make one's own, from wheat of known provenance.

The bread should be made as coarse as possible, for, as with all cooking, one of the aims of breadmaking is undoubtedly to make it easier to eat more than one could otherwise.

Pastry, homemade with wholemeal flour and good vegetable oil, thinly worked out and as lightly baked in the oven as possible, avoiding overbrowning, has probably been over-maligned.

Vegetarian 'meats', whose basis is often cheap peanut meal, and various industrialized food additives, can be better made at home, with lentils or soya as a base and wholemeal flour and nuts as a padding.

Yeast. The yeasts are present everywhere, and play an active and important role in the human alimentary tract, providing some of the B vitamin requirements when a fermentative flora prevails. But different yeasts produce many thousands of different nitrogenous substances, some of which are suspect. Moulds, close relatives of yeasts, are known to manufacture some of the most deadly chemicals, such as the cancer producing substances in mouldy peanut meal. While fresh fruit and bakers yeasts are probably excellent, care should be taken with brewers yeast, and only small amounts consumed. As for the so called hydrolized yeast preparations, made from disintegrating yeast cells usually in a strongly salted medium, they are definitely suspect. Their content of the B vitamins may be high, but they also contain nitrogenous extractives and other substances which have a dramatic effect on the blood-forming system, too dramatic not to be harmful.

The seeds of the leguminous plants

Green peas and beans when fresh are close to other green vegetables and are excellent, but pulses are in some cases suspect. A few contain lethal amounts of hydrocyanic acid. Two which appear to pass the test are lentils and soya beans. Raw peanuts are barely edible. Cooked when fresh they might pass, but a tropical crop, whose storage conditions are never known by the consumer, they are a very suspect food item in view of the extremely dangerous mould products they may harbour.

It is of great interest that a milk substitute for infants made from soya beans is now available which appears to meet all the needs of the developing infant. Mothers who are not able to breast feed for a sufficient time, should seriously think of such substitutes rather than condemn their offspring to a start in life which entails a permanent handicap to their arteries for which cow's milk is probably responsible.

Coconut. These can be obtained today in fairly fresh condition, and are an excellent food. Human milk fats are closer to those present in 'coconut milk' than to those of cow's milk. A host of attractive preparations can be made from the dried meal.

Sugar. The evil of sugar is that it fools the call of sweetness for fruits. The common belief that brown sugar is preferable, indeed beneficial, is unfounded, for the brown is due to caramelization and to metallic contamination in the course of manufacture. The content of B vitamins, not derived from the plant juices but formed as molasses is stored before the sugar is separated from it, is not sufficient justification. It is curious to observe that in the days when hygiene was all the craze, white sugar, like white flour and white rice were thought of as better than the brown products because they were cleaner and purer, today there has been a reversal into an equal absurdity, when anything 'brown' is necessarily good.

82

Honey, another cult food, honey is designed for extremely rapidly growing insects, not humans. Although 'natural', there is no reason to suppose that it is preferable to sugar. There is, alas, no way out; if humans want sweet things while remaining healthy, they should have fruits.

Mushrooms, fungi. There he goes again, the reader will say, belittling the one gourmet article of the vegetarian! But the aim is to face the facts, point out the extremely thin line of normality; it is up to the individual to decide how far he will swerve from the line, how much he is willing to pay for the deviant pleasures. The fact is that primates are as innately terrified by the sight of a mushroom, as by that of a spider or a snake! Although only a few fungi kill, most, if not all, cause various subtle sensitivity reactions in a majority of people. Commercially grown mushrooms are increasingly subjected to a rain of chemicals. However, if one comes upon a lucky patch of bluits, chanterelles, or capes, it would amount to cowardice to resist them.

Leafy foods. As already indicated, it is not the more mature leaves, but the tender shoots which are intended to feature in moderation in the human diet. Since these are scarce, population pressure has encouraged the use of harder leaves, like the brassicas, which usually need cooking. It is not therefore surprising that various contradictions have been discovered. The brassicas, for instance, contain substances which interfere with thyroid function. The already mentioned poisonous oil, from rape seed, is the product of a member of that plant family. They should therefore be looked upon as emergency rather than regular foods.

Members of the lettuce family, the cruciferae such as the cress, and many other tender green leaves, appear satisfactory. A neglected green food is the tender green shoots of grass.

Onions and garlic. Both contain extremely irritating and toxic substances which can induce serious anaemias and in large amounts, can possibly be fatal. They also often result

83

in hypersensitivity reactions of the mucosae and skin, and in some people appear to affect the mind, inducing lethargy and stupour. They should only be used sparingly.

Roots, tubers. Here also, the ability to be eaten raw is a good test, which allows carrots, and celeriac to pass, while casting doubt on many others. Those members of the mustard family with roots, such as radish, contain strong irritants and are suspect.

Tropical fruits. Many people who have lived in the tropics have become upset from eating tropical fruits, or at least developed a certain antipathy for particular fruits, longing for the more temperate apple. It is the high growing fruits which are usually involved. The ground living prehumans would not have had ordinary access to them. An example known to contain toxic substances, injurious to the liver, is the Avocado. It has surprisingly been found to induce mastitis in mammals! Another is the mango, beautiful, but frequently nauseating and containing a milk which tends to irritate the lips and mouth. Low growing tropical and semi-tropical fruits, on the other hand, such as the banana, the pineapple, the citrus family, are pleasant and wholesome. But many attractive low growing berries and fruits of tropical regions are also extremely poisonous.

Man's ideal dietary can evidently be extended, but care is needed, for many things commonly consumed and lightly assumed to be wholesome and good turn out to be suspect. Even beauty and attractiveness are no longer a reliable guide when one moves into an environment very different from that of one's genetic wombing, or is exposed to apparently edible products from a foreign environment. Evidently, many foods which carry a relatively light risk, such as the potato, have a role as an emergency item, and at the present, the entire planet is in an emergency. But even if one is likely to be obliged to trespass the narrow limits of the ideal set by the very particular perimeters of humanization, one should at least appreciate how extremely narrow these limits happen to be, and realize that a levy is inevitable for the common sloppy and insensitive approaches to eating. Those coming the closest to the ideal human diet are the vegans, and, somewhat less close, the vegetarians. These people are usually above average in sensitivity, in an awareness of self and of others, of things and creatures, which is one reason why many of them come to differ from the common patterns in the first place. There can be no doubt that the subjective rewards are considerable, providing a sense of compassion and purpose, a zeal for what is whole and natural, and a delight in simplicities, rarely met in the general modern confusion. It is this cleansing of the doors of perception which no doubt accounts for the fact that many of the more sensitive people in the arts are attracted to vegetarianism while the more tough minded tend to go in an opposite dionysian direction of booze and beef.

One does find in the ranks of vegetarians persons with a tendency to anxiety neurosis above the usual, as one does in any sensitivity demanding pursuit. Their condition is usually improved or cured, thanks to the sense of purpose and an effective life-pattern and idealism which vegetarianism can provide. But there are the few health-kick vegetarians who may not rise beyond a self-centred preoccupation. If that was all there was to vegetarianism, it would be a shallow concern, even if the pursuit of health is a primordial duty.

The great advantage of vegetarianism today is not only its practice, but the philosophy it offers regarding other human beings, living creatures and nature generally. As the help in these directions which past religions could provide is now minimal, vegetarianism is particularly well suited to offer a life-pattern ideally adapted to modern conditions, restoring a sense of purpose and participation in the natural world, without which human beings are only too obviously alienated and distraught, the reason probably why an increasing number of young are being attracted to the vegetarian ideology.

With regards the bodily advantages, one can be less definite. In the first place, some people become vegetarians as a result of chronic ill-health, when all else has failed, a fact which tends to falsify any comparative study. It is a sad fact that many people are congenitally less robust than others, disadvantages all too often intensified by wrong feeding in infancy and childhood. Such people are certain to be better off as vegetarians, but they may remain handicapped compared with the more genetically robust, living so called normal lives.

But vegetarianism by itself may not be enough. A person giving up meat and fish but indulging in eggs and dairy produce may be no better off. Indeed, it is possible that a person having some lean meat and fish, but no eggs and dairy produce, would be less exposed to the long-term disasters of cholesterol, saturated fats and uric acid, what ever other insidious physical and mental effects attend. Vegetarian children eating the usual amounts of sweets, jams and sugar have teeth in every way as bad as the general population.

As already mentioned, veganism without a supplement of vitamin B_{12} is dangerous. With this supplement, it is probably as close as one can get to the ideal human diet, but perhaps for economic réasons, fruits may not feature sufficiently. It is probably as far as one can get practically in avoiding the usual long-term infirmities, gout and arthritis, colds and constipation, and the common afflictions of daily living. This should also apply to vegetarians, provided a sufficiency of uncooked foods and fruits is the rule.

In this context, the importance of activity cannot be overemphasized. The human body, and mind, are only optimally adaptable in terms of a certain pattern of activity. This pattern must have been originally set by the demands of ground living and food-gathering, and has certainly not changed since, no matter how sedentary human beings have become in urban conditions. This pattern is characterized, not by bursts of violent activity, but rather by prolonged moderate activity. For a ground-living primate to be able

FOOD FIT FOR HUMANS

to fulfil its environmental and social obligations, would demand at least the equivalent of three hours walking a day. Medicine has now realized the importance of this kind of activity, of the risks of inactivity to the heart, as those of excessive activity which entails athletism, or the weekend violent games of tennis or squash. One must insist, that no matter how ideal the diet, optimal physiological conditions will not be met unless this basic activity pattern is simultaneously met. Life must simply be arranged to meet it, an arrangement facilitated by the energy crisis.

There are the half-hearted vegetarians, keen on keeping in with the 'normals' in their smoking and drinking habits and not averse to some meat and fish occasionally, 'for social reasons'. Such people are often less well than most, the victims of fatigue, of disturbed sleeping and of petty inconveniences, which should not be the lot of vegetarians. The high levels of protein and vitamin B complex on a mixed dietary do undoubtedly protect, to some extent, from the damage of alcohol and other poisons. Vegetarians, particularly those living on largely refined cereal foods, using sugar, are very vulnerable. Although very moderate amounts of non-distilled drinks like cider, beer and the lighter wines, are probably beneficial when consumed in the right circumstances, as we shall see, vegetarians are not equipped to keep up with common bad habits.

People who become vegetarian in later life often do so as the result of some dire warning or health disaster for which medicine can do little or nothing. Usually, such a change of diet brings much benefit, but it would be expecting too much to suppose that the unbiological trespass of many years can be completely annulled. It is the young who especially benefit from a vegetarian diet, the best possible assurance that the developing tissues of brain and body are formed under the most ideal conditions. To cut out breast feeding, and to feed infants on animal foods, is not only likely to lead to mental disquiet, but, in maturity, to a higher incidence of degenerative disease.

15. Beautiful People, Beautiful Things

The Creation is a whole, all isolation is disintegration. In the making of the human, nature has attained its highest expression of wholeness, in love, in the pursuit of beauty, order and harmony. But for the wholeness of the human condition to be attained, a wholeness in all things contributing to human existence is indispensable. The importance of food to life in general emphasizes its supreme importance in the attainment of human wholeness, and only a highly specific pattern of eating can meet this highest achievement of evolution.

Mankind on this planet has been the unfortunate victim of terrible times and tribulations. Barely had humanization been achieved, than the earth underwent a prolonged period of intermittent and devastating glaciation, with world-wide repercussions. During these terrible times, human beings were obliged to adopt ways of living in order to survive which departed widely from the human ideal previously set by nature. Although when the Ice Ages subsided some ten thousand years ago, the majority of human beings tended to resume ways of living more tolerably human, inventing agriculture in the process to ward against further catastrophe, many bad habits have persisted, particularly regarding feeding, which, as we have suggested, accounts in large part for the horrors and abnormalities of human behaviour.

Many parts of the world today should be sympathetic to a properly human condition, but because of the importance of cortical conditioning, these bad habits persist and remain

88

a most dehumanizing influence, responsible for the terrors of human existence and the ugliness of the environment. As the means of expressing anger and hatred against nature, against other creatures, against man himself have increased with the industrial age, so nature has become increasingly soiled and desecrated, and man's chronic inhumanity to man has become more sharpened. The situation is critical, for every aspect of the contemporary crisis examined shows a course set on annihilation and extinction. If further appeals to reason, to science, to politics, to sociology, to economics are certain to be frustrated unless backed by a genuine change of heart, so are the more simpleton calls for a return to nature, for a denial of civilization. Man is too wounded and humiliated a creature, too complicated by culture to be able to act from such purity. Salvation is likely to be very, very demanding.

The change must begin from within, important as the tangible aspects of life happen to be. One simply must first restore the belief that the human being is a noble, sacred creature, holding the most essential post in the creative enterprise of the universe. Anything less must entail alienation. Since no reasonable argument can change the colours of the soul, colour must be played, like music to the insane, in the hope that slowly, progressively, the divine sensitivities will be recovered, and the mind made whole.

Although ugliness tends to cancel the craving for beauty, wholeness and purity, to be surrounded by beauty and harmony, to practise it at every possible opportunity, must in the long run work. One has the examples of this in the arts. People are often drawn to the arts as a reaction against the puerilities and frustrations of living, the deceptions of gain and material power. While artists, musicians and poets themselves are usually simple people, little good at worldly tasks, the patrons have always been people of power, in their lives ruthless and hard, yet strangely softened in the presence of the beauty and divinity of art. They are not likely to become gurus and saints as a result, but they are more whole and human for it, certainly worse without it. The sensitivities on which the arts trade should be pursued in every possible aspect of living; nothing which is not beautiful should be tolerated, whatever its apparent lures.

The aim of this book has been to emphasize that such sensitivities are eminently applicable to man's most important biological function, eating. Not only is it a matter of the choice of the right kinds of foods. The attitude towards food, the conditions under which foods are eaten can provide a most important occasion for developing an overall, humanly compatible attitude and a recovery of the sensitivities, of the meaning of being human.

This is not a new appeal. All other peoples had discovered that sacrament and myth are the supreme means of incorporating thought, feeling and action into a meaningful human cosmology. One finds, among primitives, as among other less materialistically preoccupied civilizations, that nothing is left out. All is made hallowed, meaningful and sacred. Part of the tragedy of the West, thanks to misinterpretation of the significance of science to society, has been to purge life of mythical meaning. Eating is an excellent opportunity to restore this indispensable strategy.

How one eats is as important as what one eats. Eating cannot be a matter only of belly filling, of meeting calories, proteins, and the other dietary essentials, but the daily recurring opportunity to express joy, to contemplate beauty, to feel the craving for purity, and, a need particularly ignored today, to feel and express gratitude for the bounties of the earth. All peoples and ages have in fact insisted that food should be communally partaken, making it a socially bonding ritual, a bodily function raised to a high social and spiritual level, becoming in the process a joyful sacrament enacting the glory and joy of life.

After all, food is not an incidental occurrence. It is the product of a quite fantastic creative ecology on the part of nature, which began some fifteen thousand million years ago, and has been ever since groping for the expression of the inherent drive for harmony, beauty, and creativity in all matter, ever more explicit, until its culmination in the human being. As we have seen, the beauty of fruits and flowers, of all things humanly good, reflect this deep goading at work in all nature. Unless these qualities had found previous expression in fruit and flower, the human mind would have been an impossibility. In spite of the apparent fumblings and distractions of time, of the long haul of evolution, seen with the unitive vision of gods, man finds a summit place in the operations of Creation. As an important constituent in this realization, such a providential offering as food should be partaken in joy, and in humility and reverence, a thanksgiving to the gods and powers responsible for this strange and wonderful place.

The right kind of attitude to nature, to food, indeed to all whole, natural things is best illustrated in Zen practice, which teaches that loose, unconnected thinking is necessarily bad, while at the same time it insists that a rigid, imposed direction, the kind favoured by the puritans and fascists, is also bad. Living is a constant juggling for which every occasion becomes an opportunity of practice, every thought, every touch, every sight, and especially every act.

How can this apparent contradiction be resolved in ordinary living? By sensing the inherent sanctity, dignity and cosmic connection of all that is worthy of human doing. Then, in the simple outfolding of such an act, no matter how elemental and superficially trivial, a sense of profound, exquisite meaningfulness results, beyond all analysis and doubt. This can be practised in virtually any aspect of living, in one's daily work, in one's relations to others, in the contemplation of nature, in the arts, in sport, in some particular hobby. Eating is an excellent opportunity for so doing, which raises the simple act to a high order, physically and spiritually enhancing, and providing a level of satisfaction and joy beyond verbal description.

Zen is not native to the European mind and tradition, and such a suggestion will at first seem esoteric. Yet many people do in fact attempt to practise what is being suggested in their daily lives, having discovered intuitively that it is the best course through the jungles of civilized confusion and uncertainty. Many artists, for instance, are Zen practitioners without realizing it, finding an integration and joy in their creative procedures which is pure Zen. The fact is that with a modicum of desire, what is being suggested is quite easily realizable, and all the more easily in the pursuit of a natural dietary.

This exercise can begin with the preparation of food, through its presentation and serving, to consumption, stages necessarily demanding familial and social participation. Evidently, the environment becomes of great importance. One should forgo eating rather than eat in squalid, ugly surroundings. Joyful, enticing, uplifting conversation, music and periods of quiet and meditation should be an intrinsic aspect of the pattern. By contrast, the usual futile banter, the ribald and mischievous exchanges of usual entertainment show themselves up as a counter strategy to deny the humanizing relevance of the meal, one more aspect of the subtle and all-permeating impoverishment of the sensitivities.

Regular meal times constitute a device for the convenience of cooks and the cortical conditioning to greed. Meals should be left to the kind of intuitive communal decisions one finds children displaying in their games.

Eating can undoubtedly induce a 'high', an ecstatic type of experience, of the kind one can derive in the most humanizing raptures of life, in love, in communion with nature, in art, and, as every age and culture has discovered in its own ways, through certain drugs. Although it has become so rare and out of line with the materialistic pursuit of modern society, hence the recourse to drugs, it is a natural and most normal human experience, one which the more humanistic and benign primitives appear to enjoy throughout the waking day and in their dream ecstasies also. It comes, as a more or less continuous irradiation of joyfulness, of a sense of profound relevance and belonging, with peaks amounting to rapture, as the reward for life wholly and humanly lived, for effective social and communal compassion and service, for sexual love achieved as for the extensions of loving freed of all sexuality; it comes in the practice of any humanly enhancing occupation, of work shared and socially relevant, of art, of ritual, of religion.

The essential characteristic of the 'high' experience, as of the 'high' dream, is that the level of experience is so altered that ordinary verbal descriptions and analyses are pointless. Its only possible evidence is its experience, which is the reason why it has become so neglected in a materialistic culture which has increasingly insisted that only the solid material things are real. But although rarely experienced by the majority of people today, except perhaps for the common intense intimations of puberty and of youth, it can be easily recovered, so well as to become the most rewarding ingredient in living.

Food appears to have a singular capacity for inducing such a 'high'. No doubt this can be entirely due to the sacramental element in eating, with its profound humanizing associations, but there could also be a more physiological boosting to it. The attractiveness, beauty and purity of natural foods are such a boosting, for the 'high' experience is necessarily a hyper-aesthetic experience. Ugliness is anathema to it.

In another book, the writer mentioned an observation of Macacus monkeys in the wild, in a drunken, rapturous condition following feasts on ripe guavas. So keen were they on the effects, that some individuals were seen to prefer the overripe fallen fruits to those on the bough. Is this a perversion, or does it reflect a natural boost to the joy of living which primate eating is intended to provide? An analysis of ripe guavas revealed the interesting fact that they contained up to 0.8 per cent ethyl alcohol, while those on the ground could have as much as 2 per cent to 3 per cent.

Because of its crude abuses as a mind-fuddling drug in

the West, entailing the consumption of large amounts of alcoholic drinks, alcohol is a misunderstood substance. When very small amounts of alcohol are taken, *in the right frame of mind*, it is nothing but a stimulant of the higher, humanizing emotions. It is only when this threshold is exceeded that alcohol passes quickly from being a stimulant, to a depressant, cutting out the higher aspects of mental functioning and thus inducing a lower, frequently subhuman level of experience and behaviour. The importance of the right frame of mind has been observed in the case of other psychotropic substances. Taken without the uplifting influence of sacrament, they have banal and frequently antihuman results. Taken in a sacramental atmosphere, they can be potently humanizing.

The humanly enhancing effects of minimal amounts of alcohol taken in a sacramental context was not missed by the early Christians. Some early sects so managed to enhance the quite minimal amounts of alcohol taken in the sacrament that they would dance and shake with divine rapture, to the point of becoming scathingly called the 'shakers' by those who did not share their rapture.

The fact that yeasts specialized for converting sugar into alcohol are present on the skins of all fruits, that naturally such fruits become bruised, if ever so minutely as by the effects of wind, would imply that any creature designed to live preponderantly on fruits would necessarily partake of certain minimal amounts of alcohol. Knowing how canny nature, in the guise of natural selection, happens to be in making use of any such offerings, it is reasonable to suppose that such minute traces of ethyl alcohol were made use of in the human genesis to act as a stimulant to the higher humanizing faculties. If a 'high' experience is a humanly decisive experience, then such a stimulation would have been as much a tool in humanization as the perception of order and beauty in nature, as the evolution of the musical capacities of the human voice. It would have been an ideal antidote to the risks of the antihuman substances which can, as we have seen, arise in the course of deviant dietaries. Granting the relatively large amounts of fruits intended to be eaten, enough alcohol could be derived to induce the kind of 'high' described, emphasizing the humanizing role of food in general.

There are hints that in prehistory, such feasting occurred, and that the grape, a typical low growing fruit of EuroAsia, featured in such feasts. But with the advent of the Ice Ages, or the ending of the first great Interglacial during which humanizing conditions applied, a disturbed environment led to a disturbed way of life. It was not a big step unfortunately for the minimal amounts of alcohol in natural foods to give way to the higher amounts made available in especially fermented fruits, in accord with the rising sub-human arousals of a disturbed existence. So the fermented juices of fruits became linked to the Dionysian cults; as innocence was lost, so these evidently became more orgiastic and lascivious. Quite early in human history alas, alcohol became an active agent in dehumanization, as it still is.

To say that beauty goes with health, and that health is the reward of wholeness, requires a definition of beauty distinct from its usual sexy involvements. Necessarily natural beauty is designed to enshrine sexual love, but this is different from the beauty, which is no more than a veiled invitation to licence, evident in entertainment, in fashion, in the novel, in a romanticized sexuality not so far from embellished pornography. Natural beauty demands purity, and is inseparable from love. In the eyes of love, provided there is no untoward blemish, what could be seen as sexually plain could appear as of great beauty, a matter of internal light rather than of outward provocation, of wholeness rather than surface. That the human being, when truly human, is particularly attuned to this definition of beauty is made evident in art. Indeed, when it is the 'sexy' kind of beauty that prevails, one has not to do with art, but with pornography.

It is a fact, which anyone can put to the test, that a return

95

to a natural dietary not only restores health, but beauty as just defined. The foul breath, and humiliating body odours, supporting a vast artificial industry, give way to a natural sweetness. It is remarkable how fragrant the skin becomes on such a diet. The common greasy patches on forehead and nose, the dilated pores and psoriasis, the crinkly piggy fat and sagging which deform give way to a clarity, a firmness and a harmony of movement even in long abused bodies, and the eyes, those true portals to the soul, become bright and alive. There is enough evidence to sustain hope, that even advanced so called incurable disease can yield to a natural restoration, particularly when this is accompanied by a supporting restoration in human faith.

But sadly, in some of the most terrible ills against which all the skills of medicine and science remain largely powerless, the cancers and mutilations of ageing, mostly the results of human mischief and misunderstanding of nature, the body has no experience of reaction and defence. Death must then come, and be faced, as it must anyway, however joyful and wonderful life has been. In a civilization geared to the worship of material power, death is a most terrifying, utterly humiliating event. As nothing but an animal, knowing only material things, death is totally unacceptable, and those who say that they have resigned themselves to it on such terms, have in truth only shut their eyes to its ultimately humiliating power. Contemplating the wholeness and progressive achievements of life, it would be a contradiction of the entire enterprise of Creation to produce a creature aware of itself, and so of death, without some compensatory adaptation. Such compensations have perennially come in the form of a transcendental belief that the human being is not entirely in bondage to time and space, a belief lost in the present crisis of materialism. It will have to be restored, if human beings are to recover a dignified and meaningful place in the Creation. There is no reason why it should not be a perfectly natural restoration. There are pointers today even in science that so called material reality is much more than space, time and substance. But while this is at present a challenge for the individual to face for himself, nature has equipped the human to face death, in making death itself the culminating 'high' to living. Even following the terrible and prolonged torments of disease, there is abounding evidence that death can come as an ecstasy, although it would seem that the 'high' of dying is more likely to be the reward for a life lived wholly and in respect of natural law.

Just as there is a natural way to living, so there is a natural way to dying, one completely ignored by the modern age, one in fact actively rejected by the medical profession. It is a simple way, practised by all other cultures. At the end of a long life humanly lived, the intimation of death comes with a kindness that robs it of fear. On the contrary, there is a welcome and a reassurance about it. When death comes sooner, shortcutting the natural span, death can still be met by a letting go, when all hope is gone, by simply fasting out. For those who have regularly practised the fast in the course of living, there will be the reassurance that this simple act brings with it intimations of transcendence, of purity and glory which thoroughly defy the apparent finality of material things. Fasting out implies abandoning the sacrament of eating for the sacramental act of dying. The same hallowing, reverential, grateful approach is needed, the same envelopment in beauty, joy and purity. The timeless association of the human and the floral should not follow, but precede death; flowers should be for the dying, not for the dead, the reminder in such wonderful things, that nature is profoundly humanly attuned, and that wherever the Creation goes, there will its chosen creatures, in rapturous joy and fulfilment, go also.

16. Hints for the Millennium

In happier times, fruits and salads feature more predominately in the dietary, just as they go out in darker times. The head gardener of James II, was of the opinion that an ordinary salad should have at least 30 ingredients (mentioned in the *Popular Encyclopaedia of Gardening*, by H. H. Thomas and G. Forsyth). The tender roots of daisy, of fennel, of angelica and campion, as well as of carrot and parsnip were used. Leaves of wild and cultivated plants, whose names are likely to sound foreign to many a city-dweller but which abound, were also popular—dandelion, cowthistle, primrose, violet, tarragon, rocket, sage, hyssop, marigold, marjoram, leek tops, purslane, cowslip, basil, borage, chevil, daisy, vine and marrow tendrils, sorrel, scurvy grass, broom and elder buds and many other things, procurable without cost by the diligent. Flowers were also added liberally, those of dandelion, angelica, nasturtium, rose, primroses, etc. The happy Elizabethans were especially fond of salads, and seldom had a meal without one.

Just as fruits should be available at all times, the humanizing decoration in every room, in every office, and eaten whenever desired, so the salad should form the artistic focus of every meal. As John Evelyn, the salad authority of the seventeenth century remarked, the picking and preparing of salads is a great and legitimate art, giving much pleasure and healthfulness in its practice.

If one has no back garden, many things can be grown from seeds in boxes, from the common 'mustard and cress' to the germinating shoots of cereals, of wheat, barley, maize. If you buy or are given roses, eat one! If you are lucky in having something of a garden, or access to a growable patch, there is no limit to your contribution to health and joy. Many vegetables allowed to flower make beautiful flowers, e.g., the Jerusalem Artichoke, which, incidentally, is delicious grated raw with olive oil, giving very much less wind than when cooked. This is true regarding the artichoke as well. There are few more beautiful flowers than the enormous nettle of the artichoke. Cardoons are easier to grow in England than artichokes proper. The hearts are delicious raw, and the leaves can be wrapped with newspaper and blanched, the tips eaten raw and the rest cooked as a delicious vegetable.

To extend the role of fruits, when they are scarce or expensive, the 'rawcost' of the Scandinavians and the Swiss can be resorted to. The principle is to batter the fibres of the harder parts of roots and leaves so as to make them approach the softer consistency of fruits, enabling them thereby to be eaten in the larger quantities needed for meeting the needs of vitamin C and bulk generally. Although this can be done by hand chopping and macerating, there are many mechanical gadgets which save much time.

As earlier mentioned, one should not become geared to a fixed pattern of eating in a family; even in entertaining, spontaneity can be left greater opportunities, and meals should be joyfully prolonged with long intermittences— many courses need be no more than attractive snippets! It is however usually more convenient to prepare the day's eating after a breakfast of cereal, fruit and light tea or herbal. The main meal is best taken during the day, not late at night. For those working, fruits and bread and spread can be taken during the day, and the main meal taken on returning, followed by exercise and recreation. Later in the evening, a warmed soup, a light vegetable dish or a cooked fruit pudding should be sufficient.

The main meal should begin with fruits or rawcost, and

99

end with them; the salad dish should be laid as the centre-piece, available to be dipped into while the other courses are eaten. On a natural diet, one barely needs to drink at meals. It is ill-conceived to drink large amounts of commercial fruit drinks during meals. If wine is taken on festive occasions, it is not a bad idea to dilute it, and prepare it as a wine cup, with various herbs, rather than drinking it neat.

A day on fruits is a splendid idea. Once a week should suffice, but if one begins to feel jaded, irritable, tired, or at the first tremors of a cold, of an ache, then one should go on fruits, and stay on fruits for several days if necessary. If one is unwell, the quantity of fruits should be cut down, and fruit juices, adequately diluted, taken instead. In more severe disease, nothing but diluted fruit juice should be taken. Except in chronic overfeeding or advanced degenerative disease, anything more than a short fast is not recommended.

In looking through the recipe books, one can pick those needing the least cooking, just as one can usually leave out the more questionable items like eggs, substituting by a flour sauce, or nut or lentil padding. Undue cooking can be avoided by soaking. For instance, if rice is soaked for 24 hours, it needs little more than a few minutes simmering. A tasty risotto can be prepared from such rice, by adding finely chopped raw items, onions, garlic, tomatoes, and other vegetables, sprinkled with grated nuts. Those who cannot have their cereals firm, owing to chewing troubles, can further break down soaked grains in a blender.

Lentils, soya and other hard grains and seeds, can be similarly soaked, up to 48 hours and more, acquiring in the process a delicious sweetness. Thus soaked, lentils will cook adequately in ten minutes simmering. A useful thickening is provided by semolina, obtainable for making gnocci in several grain sizes. Added to soaked lentils, mushed cereals or soyas, and lightly cooked, a sufficiently solid mixture results, which can be used either 'sour', with vegetables and spices, or 'sweet', with fruits, or dried fruits. A flour sauce is

100

also useful, obtained by stirring sufficient wholemeal flour in oil, cold, to make a creamy paste, followed by gentle heating for two or three minutes, followed by adding water, vegetable juice or skimmed milk. Sour milk can also be used, the curds resulting beaten down to form a uniform mixture. For a change, wine or cider can be used. Cold or warm sauces, with infinite varieties of taste, can be prepared by making this mixture more dilute.

Do not skimp on uncooked oil; pour it liberally on foods. The human love of fat is really a love of soft fat, of oil, first relished in mother's milk, and later in the oil plentiful in the germ of seeds and cereals. It helps to keep the tissues firm and young.

Much harm is done by the popular recipes for slimming, usually recommending an increase in unnatural foods like meat, and cutting down on essential human foods like cereals, fruits and oil, with the result that as one becomes more lean, so one becomes more toxic, twisting a few more of the spirals of the degeneracies which will ripen in old age. Body fat is indispensable for health, for the proper support of organs as for a normal reserve of energy which the body is designed to carry. But as every farmer knows, a fact apparently ignored by most human nutritionists, one can decide the kind of fat laid down by the kind of fat eaten, soft or crinkly, streaky or hard. Saturated fats, the fats in all animal foods, lay down hard fat in the tissues, which deforms the normal aesthetic lines of organs and limbs, and accounts for the ugly deformities, layerings and bulges of even quite young people today. Hard fat further damages the cells in which it is laid.

The soft fat laid down from vegetable oils does not deform in this way, unless grossly abused, and even then the limbs tend to remain smooth, the bulges not necessarily ugly. There is a sexual difference in the way fat accumulates. Male sex hormone has a specific effect on metabolism generally, helping to keep the body lean, an indispensable condition for healthy, efficient muscles, a male prerogative. When the male sex hormones wane with age, wisdom would decree that the level of eating should decrease. It is usually the reverse that applies, resulting in the monstrous deformities of a majority of ageing civilized males. The female hormones, on the other hand, encourage the deposition of fat on those areas of maximal erotic appeal, the breasts, the hips and buttocks, sites, alas, readily sabotaged by overfeeding. The predilection for skinny women, as now prevails in the fashion world, is probably a homosexual de-feminization of women.

Of greater concern to aesthetics, soft fat is easily mobilized and removed from the depot tissues, while hard fat, once laid down, can be very difficult to remove in a synchronized manner that leaves the body aesthetically whole. Even after prolonged dieting, it tends to remain in the weary sagging tissues in the backwater areas where circulation is the poorer, particularly the belly and hips. The reason is that the space left as soft fat is mobilized, is rapidly filled up, as the healthy, elastic protoplasm bounces back into shape. But owing to the damage done to the cells by hard fat, elasticity is lost, so that the spaces left become filled with water. This can persist for a long time, accounting for the fact that weight loss on dieting appears so slow, and, what is even more frustrating, as soon as a 'normal' diet with fat is resumed, these spaces become rapidly occupied by fat again.

Few subjects are so confused as that of dieting, of overweight, in which an absence of any notion of normality is apparent at every turn. Undoubtedly, when overweight is due to hard fat eating, it is a killer. Soft fat, unless in considerable excess, is probably less dangerous. There is evidence that the incidence of circulatory and heart diseases is significantly less in the overweight Italian emigré communities in the States, living largely on pasta and much vegetable oil, than in the community generally. The real test of adequate or excess adiposity is the resulting aesthetics or inaesthetics. When fat, even soft, becomes unattractive, it is bad without further question.

Exercising the body daily should be a pleasure, not the

punishment it often becomes in the various cult systems. If one cannot walk sufficiently daily—two or three hours—then on several occasions during the day one can ambulate joyfully, wherever one happens to be, alone or communally, with music or without, in freedom and abandon, going through the kind of natural movements one would naturally perform as a native food gatherer—reaching for imaginary apples, bending to pick imaginary berries, thrusting, raising, bending, jumping, dancing, jogging.

Evidently one should take up this kind of spontaneous exercising of the entire body, eye and mind in the ways to which it has been adapted through millions of years of evolution, progressively, all the more carefully and gently the longer one has remained a sedentary, indolent victim of urbanism. People with heart trouble should not try them at all, and if any malaise is felt while doing them, one should stop immediately, and rest. Pleasure, a sense of enhancement of vitality, a burst of joy in living, are the assurances that all is well.

The proper balance to exercise is relaxation, not a sedentary fidgeting, a tense, anxious stationary restlessness which most people understand by 'doing nothing'. The natural ability to relax, a letting go rather than a concentrated effort, is so far lost, that it must be diligently practised in order to be recovered. One can start in a small way, relaxing the fingers, then the hand, then the arm, and progressively the entire body. Once acquired—it cannot be consciously imposed—the mind itself is predisposed, the electric patterns of the brain change, and it can even become possible to affect the Birger rhythms, the heart beat, the blood pressure in a favourable direction. Breathing is a key way of obtaining this desirable state, but the popularly advocated 'deep breathing' can be unpleasant, even dangerous, when undertaken in the usual anxious, agitated state of mind. Over-breathing, by washing out too much carbon dioxide from the blood, can produce alarming panic symptoms. Deep breathing, gently, harmoniously, slowly, should therefore only be practised when an initial ability to relax muscularly has been reached. On the other hand, eye relaxation can be beneficially practised from the start—head back to increase drainage in the anterior chamber of the eye, sitting or lying in a relaxing position, in quiet or listening to soft music, to poetry, the eyes closed, while the muscles of the lids are increasingly relaxed, so that often one reaches a condition when the eyes are half closed, without any effort. One can think of pleasant things, or attempt to cut out stray thinking altogether, to think of darkness, of colour, of light, of smoke, or non corporeal things. Cutting out sound, in noisy environments, by ear-lugging during periods of relaxation or meditation, is indispensable.

The universe is a creative enterprise; in its lapses of destruction, it cannot be said to exist. So the human place in the cosmos is a creative one; all whole, human thinking is creative, and it is only when humans are properly human that they can be said to exist fully as far as the Creation is concerned. The creative attitude becomes the measure of cosmic fitness, the qualification for belonging meaningfully in the scheme of things, the only assurance against alienation. Although there are some activities patently destructive and antihuman practised in most societies, the majority of living functions and activities have a creative potential. If this is realized, it can be developed in many of the common tasks of living, in many hobbies and interests, individually and socially. But the amateur practice of some art, of any art, of any activity with an aesthetic content, is the supreme means of exercising the creative obligation. Although it is possibly more helpful to become involved in artistic expression, no matter how amateur, to be engaged in the appreciation of any art is in itself a creative experience, whether it be the simple act of reading, of listening to poetry or music, of appreciating nature, of looking at paintings or sculpture, of trying to sense the possible aesthetic content in any situation by removing the clutter and confusion, the hideous and the obstructing. By developing the aesthetic sensitivities, as this book has from the start emphasized, one becomes all the more effectively human; while this can be exercised in the most important arena of food and feeding, it should clearly become an all-reconciling life-attitude.

17. Notes and Readings

An account of the evolution and significance of the humanizing and the aesthetic sensitivities can be found in my books, *Art into* life (London 1958) and *Art as understanding* (London 1963). *Human History* (London 1954), by the great anatomist and anthropologist, Sir Elliot Smith, remains the most convincing scientific support for an Arcadian view of man, for a natural goodness and decency. The role of mother-love in the evolution of the mammals, the prelude to the humanizing sensitivities, is dealt with by F. Alverdes in his, *Social Life in the Animal World* (London 1927). See also M. Burton's, *Animal Courtship* (London 1953).

For the innate urge to beauty in matter, made evident in crystals, minerals and molecular structure, and for the resulting sustaining aesthetic theme in nature's creativity generally, in art as in mysticism, see my, *The Crystalline Theme* (Academy Books, 1975), Sir Alister Hardy's, *The Living Stream* (London 1965) is an inspired biologist's account of the aesthetics and the directiveness of evolution, culminating in the human being.

Support for the significance of the human sensitivity to beauty comes from an unexpected quarter, the renowned physicist P. A. M. Dirac, who contends in a very readable article in the Scientific American May 1963, p. 45, that beauty in a scientific theory is the best assurance to its validity. Ugly theories are wrong theories. Support for the natural sensitivities from the arts, especially poetry, and for the Arcadian view of man, come in a delightful book, *The Golden Feast*, by R. Walker (London 1952).

Scientists no longer insist that animal foods are necessary. Although it is rarely admitted that man is not properly adapted to such foods, many authorities accept that a vegetarian dietary can be quite adequate, as does the eminent pathologist Rene Dubois, in his, *Man Adapting* (Yale 1965).

Recently, the protein controversy has flared up again, with increasing insistence that previous estimates have been far too high. As Drs Miller and Payne point out (*Strategy for a hungry world*. Nature, Vol. 25, 20 Sept 1974), there is no shortage of protein for the poor peoples of the world as long as there is enough cheap cereal available. To attempt to fill the so called protein gap by increasing the availability of animal protein at the sacrifice of primary food production is illogical. P. V. Sakhatme (Nature, Vol. 248, March 1974), claims that protein standards are in excess by nearly 60 per cent. In a recent study in New Guinea, good health was found to be maintained, on essentially vegetable foods, 53 per cent less than the standards usually considered necessary. Fish was plentiful, but was not sought or eaten by the inhabitants (New Scientist, Monitor, 25 June 1973). Dr D. McLaren also criticizes the nutritionists attempts to make available more animal protein at the expense of primary cereals (Lancet, 1974).

The conclusion that the fantastic creative pilgrimage of cosmic evolution has mind as its destiny, finds support from scientists, as in Nature, Vol. 249, p. 208, 17 May 1974. See also W. H. Thorpe's *Biology, psychology and belief* (Cambridge 1962). For a combination of science and sensitivity in an approach to nature, see V. F. Weiskopf's brilliant little book, *Knowledge and Wonder* (London 1964).

Still unique as a document by a biologist, running against the popular views of bestiality and promiscuity, is H. S. Jenning's, *The Biological Basis of Human Nature* (London 1930). It is an incrimination against science and civilization that the facts, and the theme presented, have not been subsequently developed. For a more recent account of society, without the usual lip service to the hoof and claw mentality, see Lawrence D. Sahlin's, *Origin of Society, Scientific American*. 207, 48, p. 76, September 1960.

For the effects of cortical (i.e., social) conditioning on sexual behaviour, see G. S. Ford and F. A. Beach, *Patterns of sexual behaviour* (London 1965). In his *Comparative Study of Human Reproduction* (Yale 1945), C. S. Ford provides statistical evidence for a more specific affective human sexual pattern, especially in matters affecting reproduction and breeding, which is where one would expect any genetical directives to have the most relevance.

The lie to the popular (and financially rewarding) supports for man's natural aggressivity, is ably called by the anthropologist Ashley Montagu, in his, *The Direction of Human Development* (London 1957). Although the Bestial as opposed to the Arcadian vision of man was backed by most scientists in the past, today it is largely promoted by the popularizers of science, who have found a lucrative market, and an enormous journalistic support, for thus justifying the public's bestialiness, as in Robert Ardrey and Desmond Morris. The fact that this success depends on a biased sifting of facts, an often blatant extrapolation from insufficient data or from animal data inapplicable to man, as well as in a skilled misinterpretation for effect, has not been missed by the majority of serious scientists. For a discussion, see J. Lewis and B. Towers, *Naked Ape or Homo Sapiens?* (London 1972). This book also brings out the interesting suggestion that the apparent 'nakedness' of the human body is due to a transformation of the skin into an extremely sensitive emotional route, which concurs with the erotic transfiguration of the entire human body through beauty and sensitivity for the purposes of sexual love.

Quastel's work on the possibility of mind-disturbing substances formed in the human gut, is to be found in a book edited by Joseph Needham, *Perspectives in Biochemistry* (Cambridge 1937), the more recent work by S. S. Kety and others is in an article, *New perspectives in psychopharmacology*, in *Beyond Reductionism*, edited by Arthur Koestler,

P. D. McClean's, *The paranoid streak in man*, on which Koestler based his notions of a faulty evolution of the human brain, is to be found in the same book.

Kuru, a fatal disease of the Central Nervous System in humans, now known to be spread by the eating of brains by some cannibalistic tribes in New Guinea, is caused by a 'slow virus'. It has been suggested that as mental diseases are seasonal (especially schizophrenia), and as they are much more frequent in the prosperous communities, with a high standard of living, there could be a nutritional factor as well as a genetic one in mental disease (See New Scientist, Monitor, 12 July 1973).

V. Branfenbrenner's, *Origins of Alienation* (Scientific American, p. 53, August 1974) is a good account of the break between the young and the old, with its attendant social disturbances, due to disturbances in family life. The following are still worth reading, W. M. S. Russell, *The Wild Ones* (Listener, 5 Nov 1964) and his *The Affluent Crowd* (Listener, 12 November 1964).

A. Koestler, *The Ghost in the machine* (London 1967), a fascinating discourse on man's mental predicament, although his inferences are faulty. For a reappraisal of the meaning of mind in its highest aspects, see *Altered States of Consciousness*, edited by C. T. Dart (London 1958). The benefits of food restriction in mental diseases are recorded by Y. Nikolayev in Soviet Weekly, reported by New Scientist, 414, 22 October 1964. Fifteen years of starving psychiatric patients for upwards of a week resulted in dramatic improvement, even in schizophrenics. After a period of total abstinence, fruit juice, grated carrots, sour milk, nuts, vegetables, bread and honey are given. Animal foods are ruled out. A confirmatory letter regarding results in a clinic in the UK is in New Scientist, 24 December 1964.

The Nobel prizewinning biochemist, L. Pauling, is largely responsible for the flare-up of interest in vitamin C, in his much advertised claim that his family were kept free of colds by large doses of vitamin C. But Pauling has failed to sense, or admit, the wider implications of his claim, namely, that the fact that such large doses are without any toxic effects, must mean that man is perfectly adapted to them, which in turn can only mean that he is essentially a fruit-eater.

But Pauling's orthodoxy has not prevented him from being repeatedly attacked for claims regarding vitamin C usually considered as sensational. As with amply proved phenomena like telepathy, scientists, lacking an adequate world-view, find themselves emotionally compelled to deny. But man is not unique in such large vitamin C needs. The guinea-pig, a frantic gobbler of fresh green tasties, requires as much as man on a body weight basis—a child, for instance, would need 1500 milligrams daily, instead of the 200 officially recommended. (Man Li Yew. National Academy of Science, USA, Vol. 7, p. 964, 1974.)

The ever increasing wonders of vitamin C now includes claims for counteracting the cancer-inducing nitrosamides, for reducing heart attacks, for alleviating diabetes, and, latest of all, for mitigating hang-overs! See New Scientist, 12 April 1973, and 18 April 1974.

Coffee drinking doubles the risk of myocardial infarctus ('heart attacks'). No affect appeared to be associated with tea drinking (up to six cups a day). Lancet, Vol. 2, p. 1278, 1972. That does not mean that tea drinking is healthy— only that it is less harmful!

The food crisis is focussed in the Commentary in New Scientist (18 July 1974), 'Will Britain starve?' with the following conclusion: 'Perhaps the most important of all, the public must get used to the idea that it can get by with a great deal less food than it usually consumes, and that edible protein is too valuable to feed to farm livestock.'

For the disasters of pollution, of dwindling natural resources, of overcrowding, see G. Rattray Taylor's, *The Doomsday Book* (London 1970).

Rats, made to fast for one to three days a week, live longer, with a lower incidence of all causes of death, including cancer. Dr Alec Comfort concludes that by eating less, humans should be able to increase their present lifespan by 20 *per cent* to 40 *per cent* (New Scientist, 30 March 1972).

Given a wide choice and abundance of foods, rats, with much more native instinct than man, nonetheless fail to pick the right foods. On the contrary, they have a singular ability, owing to an equivalent of human greed, to pick the pattern of eating most likely to induce cancers and the other diseases of age (Nature, Vol. 250, July 1974).

A recently discovered long-living community in Ecuador, where people live frequently over the century—the record is 130 years—on a diet essentially vegetarian and with abundant fruits, is reported in New Scientist, by D. David Davies (*A Shangri-la in Ecuador* 1 February 1973). A study of a classical example, that of the Hunzas, is in Dr D. Wrench's, *The Wheel of Health* (London 1938).

For the basal needs of salt and other constituents, as well as the feats of attempted human adaptation to different environments, see P. T. Baker, J. S. Weiner, Editors of *The Biology of human adaptability* (Oxford 1966), also G. A. Harrison, J. S. Weiner, J. M. Tanner. N. A. Bannicot's *Human biology* (Oxford 1964).

A well-known researcher on the brain, Sir J. C. Eccles, in his book, *Facing Reality* (London 1970) does not find that anything discovered by science or likely to be discovered can rule out the ancient human hoping that the mind transcends the limitations of time and space. For those who assume that science and materialism have once and for all dismissed the belief in immortality, such corrections should come as a ray of light in a dark material age.

There are many books of vegetarian recipes which can be consulted, picking out those which need the less manipulation and fussy cooking. In spite of perhaps overmuch cooking, W. and J. Fliess, *Modern Vegetarian Cookery* (London 1964), is well worth consulting for ideas. Also a happy little book by R. Mabey, *Food for Free* (London 1972). For a wide-ranging concern for the survival menage of vegetarianism, see Jon Wynne-Tyson's *Food for a Future* (London 1975).